Living (Well!) with Gastroparesis

Answers, Advice, Tips & Recipes for a Healthier, Happier Life

Crystal Zaborowski Saltrelli CHC

ISBN: 0615547753
ISBN 13: 9780615547756
Library of Congress Control Number: 2011917956
Sea Salt Publishing Rochester, NY

Gratitude is the memory of the heart.

–Jean Baptiste Massieu

To my fellow GPers:
Thank you for allowing me to be a part of your journey.
May this book educate, inspire, and empower you to live well with gastroparesis.

To Drs. Jean Fox, Brian Lacy, and Jim Swain:
Thank you for treating me as a person rather than a condition. Your medical expertise and personal kindness have made a tremendous difference in my ability to live well with gastroparesis.

To Mr. Rosenthal:
Your guidance and generosity have shaped the person I've become and the path my life has taken. Thank you.

To mom, dad, Jeremy, and Raymond:
You are my greatest blessings.
Thank you for your unconditional love and unwavering support.

Contents

My heartfelt gratitude to those who generously supported this work:

Gastroparesis & Dysmotility Foundation

Diane Sharma

Irene Zaremski Saltrelli

Timothy and Diana Zaborowski

Bonnie Bolton

Stacey Cowell

Barbara Johnson

Gerianne Leonard

Marta Luzim

Heather Murphy

Rick & Debbie Saltrelli

Kandra Burleson Small

Natasha Spoden

Gastroparesis Patient Association for Cures & Treatments

The Bomenka Family

Dan and Barbara Burleson

Jo Allison Henn

Samantha Farmer

Carol Pasinkoff

Jean Augustine

Rick Ahmann

Michelle Beckwith

Irene Bodle

Kim Furra

Sheri Gdula

Heather Jaffe

Anita Martino

LeAnne Miller

Karen Perry

Jodi Rennebu-Test

Linda M Ruvolo

Mollee Sullivan

Susan Sexton

Crystal Smith

Aliza Chana Zaleon

Jeremy Zaborowski

Angie Black

Sharona Goodman

David Spach Lane

Tanya Lorenz

Cheryl Morrison

Mary Rennebu

David and Karla Smith

The Tyma Family

Sarah Bertsch

Kelli Fudella

Bob Galvin

Tina Liouzis

Vaughan Merlyn

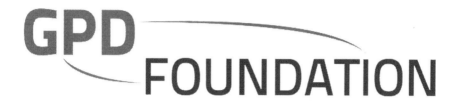

First and foremost, the GPD Foundation would like to thank Crystal Saltrelli for her dedication to and advocacy for Gastroparesis patients. She serves as a constant inspiration in the Gastroparesis community and we cannot thank her enough for her commitment and knowledge.

The GPD Foundation is working alongside Crystal Saltrelli to help Gastroparesis patients learn how to manage their symptoms and achieve a better quality of life. The ultimate mission of the GPD Foundation is to find a cure for the disease by facilitating aggressive research funding.

The GPD Foundation invites you to join us in taking action against Gastroparesis. Our vision for success is to create a community of patients, family, and friends with a common goal. Together we can make a difference for those afflicted with the disease.

For more information about getting involved in the fight against Gastroparesis, or to view our patient resources, please visit our website at **www.gpdfoundation.com**.

Sincerely,

Pamela Hoeland
GPD Foundation, President

Allie Hoeland
GPD Foundation, Executive Director

Author's Note

diet challenges

high Potassium

Diabetes

Hemochromatosis

Suppliments

Timing Medications

Sodium

blunted vili sm intestine

Introduction

Diseases can be our spiritual flat tires— disruptions in our lives that seem to be disasters at the time but end by redirecting our lives in a meaningful way.

–Bernie S. Siegel

The first time I ever heard the word "gastroparesis" was the day I was diagnosed with the condition in 2004, following a year of endless testing and doctor visits. My initial complaint had been stomach pain and what appeared to be drug-resistant acid reflux. Over time I started noticing that regardless of how hungry I was at the beginning of a meal, I felt full very quickly and was often nauseated afterward. It was a gastric emptying scan, showing "markedly delayed gastric emptying," that finally provided a diagnosis: gastroparesis.

My doctor stood in the doorway of the examining room as he offered a few vague instructions, almost as an afterthought: eat smaller meals, less fat, and less fiber. And that was it. Not even a pamphlet with more information. I left his office with a three month follow-up appointment and a whole bunch of questions. At that point I was thankful to finally have a diagnosis, but I hadn't a clue what to do about it.

I began searching for information about this seemingly rare condition. I went to the library and the book stores, but I couldn't find a single book written about the topic. I'd find a line or two here and there, but nothing that provided any real clarity or guidance. I turned to the Internet, where I found a lot of personal stories—many of which scared the daylights out of me—but still nothing to help me figure out how to feel better and live my life with gastro-paresis. I felt overwhelmed, frustrated, and alone.

Based on the doctor's vague advice, I immediately removed all high-fat foods from my diet. I switched from whole foods to processed ones that were lower in fiber. I began eating six or more small meals a day. Based on what I'd read from others online, I eventually cut out vegetables and fruits. Then I stopped eating animal protein, eggs, and cheese. Before long, I had lost nearly forty pounds, I was living on baby food and crackers, and I was more symp-tomatic than ever.

Desperate for help, I traveled with my mother to a prominent medical center in Ohio to see a specialist in motility disorders. My hopes were high as I packed my bags with a week's worth of clothes, figuring the visit would probably entail several days of testing and appointments. To my mind, I was sick, malnourished, and in desperate need of help. Unfortunately, the doctor didn't agree. After looking at my chart for about two minutes, he turned to me and said "I have patients much worse off than you. Come back when you need a feeding tube." True story.

The next few years consisted of a great deal of trial and error and consequent ups and downs. At times I felt defeated. At other times I felt hopeful. In early 2008, I was twenty-six years old, newly married, and, despite doing all I knew to do, sicker than ever. I had taken to sleeping on the couch since I was only able to actually sleep for three or four hours each night. I was in the emergency room nearly every other week because of severe pain and nausea. By that time I'd seen dozens of specialists, as well as a wide variety of alternative practitioners. I'd tried every medication available to me and spent thousands of dollars on supplements and natural remedies.

I began to realize that there wasn't a secret pill, magical diet, or all-knowing expert out there waiting to cure me of this condition. If I was going to get well, or at least *live* well, my only option was to accept that I had gastroparesis and do everything I could to better manage it. I knew that I'd have to be more proactive and become my own advocate. I knew that I needed to take better of care of myself and improve my nutrition. I finally decided that if I couldn't find the help I needed, I'd have to become the help that I needed. I wanted to learn how to start healing my body—or at least support and nourish it until modern medicine caught up with the condition.

I couldn't ignore the fact that I had to do something while I was learning these things, how-ever. I had lost nearly 50 pounds and despite the "offer" from the doctor in Ohio, I had never felt comfortable with the idea of a feeding tube. So in September 2009, having tried everything else available to me, I decided to have a gastric neurostimulator implanted at the Mayo Clinic in Minnesota. It turned out to be one of the best decisions I've ever made.

That same month, I made another life-changing decision. I started classes in holistic health and nutrition at the Institute for Integrative Nutrition (IIN). Initially, it was difficult to manage the intensive schooling while recovering from surgery. But thanks to the combination of the gastric neurostimulator and my classes, I was able to gradually make effective changes to my diet and lifestyle.

At IIN, I studied over a hundred dietary theories and learned from experts in a wide variety of disciplines. I kept what made sense for gastroparesis management and set aside what didn't. Though I started the program to help myself, it didn't take me long to realize that I had to use this information to help others, as well: to provide the guidance and support that I had been so desperate for, yet unable to find. By the time I graduated as a Certified Health Counselor, I was blogging regularly and counseling a handful of other people who had gastroparesis. I was also taking much better care of myself, improving my nutrition, and feeling physically and mentally better than I had in years.

The concepts that I learned at IIN were indispensable, but my studies there were just the beginning. As I counseled more and more clients with gastroparesis, I learned more and more about the condition. Anyone who has had gastroparesis for any length of time will tell you that everyone experiences the condition differently. While that's true in many respects, my hundreds of hours talking with gastroparesis patients revealed a great number of similarities and patterns.

It became clear to me that living well with gastroparesis wasn't just the result of finding the "right" diet or the "right" medication. It came from having a *comprehensive* management plan that included dietary modification, adequate nutrition, lifestyle practices, stress management, appropriate medical treatment, complementary therapies, and a positive attitude. That's the knowledge from which this book was born.

This is the resource that I wish I'd found after I left my doctor's office that day in 2004. I've taken everything I've learned over the past seven years, both personally and professionally, and put it all together in one place. The first half of the book is divided into seven sections, which together make up a comprehensive gastroparesis management plan. You'll find all of the information and tools that you need to become your own advocate, minimize your symptoms, improve your quality of life, and learn to *live well* with gastroparesis. The second half of the book provides you with over 75 gastroparesis-friendly recipes to use as you learn to *eat well* with gastroparesis.

You'll notice that the information is presented mostly as a Q & A. That's because I remember how many questions I had in the days, months, and years that followed the diagnosis. And I know that what most GPers want more than anything is answers to those questions: straightforward, easy-to-understand answers from someone who knows firsthand what it's like to live with gastroparesis. Along the way, I'll also share some personal stories, tips, and practical advice.

Not everything will resonate with you. Not all dietary recommendations or medical options are appropriate for everyone with gastroparesis. As you read through the book, please do as I did while studying at IIN—keep what makes sense for you and set aside what doesn't. This is *your* journey, after all. I'm just your guide.

As you read through the various sections, keep in mind that gastroparesis is not a static condition. Most of us experience variations in our symptoms and/or tolerances from day to day or week to week. For some people, symptoms resolve over time. For others, they may stay the same or worsen (though I believe that may often be a result of the chronic stress and poor nutrition that typically accompanies this condition—something you'll be taking action against by following the suggestions in this book!). It may be necessary for you to focus on or tweak various aspects of your management plan as your circumstances change over time.

If you're wondering whether *I'm* living well with gastroparesis these days, I can honestly say that I am. I still have gastroparesis but the physical symptoms are fairly well-controlled by my comprehensive management plan, which includes the gastric neurostimulator. I don't eat what most people would consider a normal diet, but I'm reasonably well-nourished and I'm able to maintain a healthy weight. Most importantly, to me anyway, I'm happy and my quality of life is quite good. I have a fantastic husband, a wonderful family, supportive friends, and a fulfilling career. My life is nothing like I imagined it would be, but I am living well and I hope that this book will allow you to say the same.

Please note that I am not a medical professional and that nothing in this book should be taken as medical advice. This book represents my opinions, based on my personal experience with gastroparesis, my education in holistic nutrition, and my work as a Certified Health Counselor specializing in gastroparesis management. My intention is not to diagnose or treat any condition; rather, it is to educate, empower, and inspire you as you learn to live (well!) with gastroparesis.

EDUCATION & SELF-ADVOCACY

What is the use of running if we are not on the right road?

–German proverb

Understanding Gastroparesis

You cannot assume that every healthcare professional you encounter will be an expert in—or even familiar with—gastroparesis. Therefore, **you** must become your own advocate. In order to be your own advocate and ensure that you're living as well with gastroparesis as possible, you *must* be well educated about the condition itself.

Part of this is the education that you're going to get from reading this book, the tools and information that you need to build your comprehensive management plan. The other part is learning what works for *you*. The first part is fairly easy—just keep reading! The second develops more slowly over time. It's a process, and you will continue to learn more about both gastroparesis in general and your own tolerances as your journey continues.

Along the way, be mindful of the sources that you're relying on for information. Take a step back and evaluate ideas before taking action. Doing too much too quickly nearly guarantees that you'll end up even more symptomatic than you started. The real key to being your own advocate is to educate yourself in a way that allows you to make conscientious decisions every day to improve your outcome.

What does gastroparesis mean?

Gastroparesis (GP) is a motility disorder in which gastric emptying is delayed. Motility refers to the contractions of the muscles within the stomach that propel food into the small intestine. If you have been diagnosed with gastroparesis, your stomach empties food more slowly than normal. While there can be motility problems in other parts of the gastrointestinal tract, a gastroparesis diagnosis applies specifically to the stomach. and meds

Is gastroparesis a disease?

Gastroparesis is considered a functional disorder. Unlike diseases that are caused by or result in visible abnormalities, you can't *see* a functional disorder upon examination or via tests such as x-rays. With gastroparesis, there is no physical obstruction or structural issue within the stomach. The problem is in the way the stomach *functions*. Specifically, the motility of the stomach is impaired. Gastroparesis is part of a group of disorders called functional gastrointestinal and motility disorders (FGIMDs).

Is gastroparesis a rare condition? It's seems like nobody's ever heard of it.

The true prevalence of gastroparesis is unknown. Estimates of the number of Americans affected by the condition range from 1.5 million to 5 million. It's likely that gastroparesis is at least as common as more widely recognized disorders like Crohn's disease and ulcerative colitis.

How is gastroparesis diagnosed?

did this

Gastroparesis is typically found after other conditions such as gastric ulcers, acid reflux, and physical obstructions have been ruled out. Sometimes your doctor may see food in the stomach during an endoscopy, despite your several hours of fasting. This is usually a clue that gastroparesis may be present. (The absence of food in the stomach during an endoscopy, however, does not rule out the possibility of gastroparesis.)

did this

The gold standard for diagnosing gastroparesis is a four-hour gastric emptying study (GES). The test is non-invasive and fairly easy for most people to complete. It involves eating a small meal, most commonly a scrambled egg and a piece of bread, which has been mixed with a small amount of radioactive tracer. Pictures are taken at regular intervals throughout the test to determine how quickly (or slowly) your stomach empties the meal.

What constitutes delayed gastric emptying?

Generally, if more than 10 percent of the test meal remains in the stomach after four hours, gastric emptying is considered delayed. Opinions may vary slightly from doctor to doctor.

My GES didn't last four hours. Is it still accurate?

Some medical facilities perform 90-minute or two-hour gastric emptying studies. In general, the four-hour test is preferred, since it's possible to have normal emptying at two hours but delayed emptying at four hours, and vice versa.

How accurate is the test overall?

While the gastric emptying study is the best tool currently available to diagnose gastroparesis, it's not a perfect test. The test provides snapshots of what happens over a few hours on one day. The problem is that gastroparesis is a dynamic condition. Gastric emptying, and therefore any symptoms, may vary from day to day or even throughout the course of the same day.

In addition, you fast for at least twelve hours before this test, and the food that you're provided is a small, low-fat, low-fiber meal (also known as "gastroparesis-friendly"). So if your stomach is emptying a gastroparesis-friendly meal too slowly, even after twelve hours of fasting, it's likely that the regular meals you're eating throughout the day empty even slower.

What's more, there's no standard version of the test, so the meal, timing and techniques used may vary widely between medical centers. This can make it difficult to interpret or compare the results of multiple studies over time or from one doctor to another.

Is it possible to get a false negative?

As I mentioned, a gastric emptying study provides a snapshot in time. It's possible that your stomach may empty more quickly on one day than it does on the next, so the results of the test may vary. Personally, I've had several gastric emptying studies over the past seven years and they've ranged from markedly delayed to nearly normal. It's also possible to have gastroparesis-like symptoms without evidence of a delay in gastric emptying. This is typically diagnosed as functional dyspepsia.

Is it possible to get a false positive (in other words, to be diagnosed with gastroparesis if I don't really have it)?

It's unlikely that a GES would show delayed gastric emptying if it wasn't present. However, a finding of delayed gastric emptying doesn't necessarily indicate an illness. Certain medications, for example, can delay gastric emptying.

How do I know if I have mild or severe gastroparesis?

The term gastroparesis only denotes that gastric emptying is delayed. It does not indicate the severity of the delay nor does it take into account the severity of the symptoms, both of which can vary dramatically among people diagnosed with gastroparesis (GPers).

Note that while many doctors will make a diagnosis of gastroparesis whether gastric emptying is 10 percent delayed or 90 percent delayed, others reserve the term for severely impaired motility. This ambiguity is why some patients may be diagnosed as having gastroparesis by one doctor and functional dyspepsia by another. The term "functional dyspepsia" is sometimes used to describe gastroparesis-like symptoms in the absence of a marked delay. It's likely that gastroparesis and functional dyspepsia, which have similar symptoms and treatment strategies, fall along the same continuum. The distinction between them is often fuzzy.

The doctor said that I have mild gastroparesis, but my symptoms seem severe. How can that be?

While delayed emptying of the stomach is the basis of a gastroparesis diagnosis, the degree of the delay does not always correlate with the severity of the symptoms experienced. For example, diabetic patients may have grossly delayed emptying but few symptoms other than the inability to adequately control blood sugar. On the other hand, there are many people who experience severe and unrelenting gastrointestinal symptoms despite nearly normal gastric emptying. This suggests that many of the symptoms associated with gastroparesis may be due to more than just dysmotility in some cases.

What else would cause the symptoms?

Some people with dysmotility also have visceral hypersensitivity. This means that nerves in the gut are more sensitive than normal and that physiological processes that most people don't even notice may cause pain or other symptoms. The bottom line is that gastric emptying time alone does not always accurately predict the severity of symptoms. While most motility specialists recognize this, general gastroenterologists who are not very familiar with gastroparesis may not.

I never vomit. Isn't that the main symptom of gastroparesis?

Though vomiting undigested food *can* be one of the main symptoms of gastroparesis, there are many people who have gastroparesis who never vomit. Nausea actually seems to be a more prevalent symptom. Other symptoms of gastroparesis include pain, early satiety (feeling full quickly), bloating, distension, heartburn, regurgitation, and reflux. You may experience any combination of these symptoms, but not necessarily all of them.

If I mostly have nausea now, might I start vomiting in the future?

In my experience with clients, most GPers start out primarily vomiting *or* primarily feeling nauseated, and this typically doesn't change over time. This is based solely on my personal experience and professional observations. I don't know of any scientific evidence that points one way or the other.

Is pain a common symptom of gastroparesis?

There was a time when doctors didn't think that having gastroparesis caused pain. However, both abdominal and chest pain are now recognized as common symptoms associated with the condition. Some doctors consider pain to be more representative of functional dyspepsia than gastroparesis. As I said, the distinction between the two diagnoses is often fuzzy.

As to the actual cause of the pain, while it may result from hypersensitivity in some cases, there doesn't seem to be a definitive answer.

Is severe bloating and/or belching normal with gastroparesis?

Bloating is quite common among people who have gastroparesis. Studies have found that nearly three of every four GPers report at least mild bloating and as many as one in three have severe bloating. Interestingly, studies have also found that the severity of the bloating is not related to the severity of the delay in emptying.

There's no clear answer as to exactly what's causing the bloating. For a large percentage of GPers, especially those who have had gastroparesis for several years, bacterial overgrowth may be present in the gut. Bacterial overgrowth can cause significant bloating and belching, as well as pain, malabsorption of nutrients, weight loss, and bowel changes.

Another possible cause of bloating is fermentation of food in the gut. Some people with functional gastrointestinal and motility disorders like gastroparesis may be sensitive to certain carbohydrates called FODMAPs. (See page 69). Foods high in FODMAPs may ferment in the gut, giving off gases that cause bloating and belching..

How do I know if I have bacterial overgrowth?

There are *trillions* of bacteria in our gastrointestinal (GI) tract, mostly in our colon, where they're not only normal but essential for proper bowel function. When the small intestine starts to resemble the large intestine, however, in terms of the kinds and number of bacteria present, you have what's called Small Intestinal Bacterial Overgrowth or Small Bowel Bacterial Overgrowth (SIBO or SBBO). SIBO can cause a myriad of symptoms, such as bloating, belching, pain, bowel changes, and weight loss. Because these symptoms overlap with those of gastroparesis, it can be difficult to determine whether or not SIBO is contributing to the discomfort you're experiencing.

Risk factors for SIBO include compromised GI motility and insufficient stomach acid. If you experience a significant amount of bloating after you eat, especially if you've had gastroparesis for several years, you struggle with constipation, and/or you take acid suppressing medication, you might consider talking with your doctor about SIBO. Testing is often done via a breath test, and treatment typically involves a course of antibiotics to eradicate the bacteria from the small intestine. Managing constipation, avoiding excess sugar in the diet, and normalizing stomach acid can be helpful in preventing continued overgrowth.

Are there other issues that can result from delayed emptying besides GI symptoms?

Aside from symptoms like vomiting, nausea, fullness, pain and bloating, delayed gastric emptying can lead to erratic swings in blood sugar, which often presents a significant challenge for those with diabetic gastroparesis. Gastroparesis can also interfere with the efficacy of oral medication, since the timing of emptying and absorption is unpredictable. We'll talk more about addressing these challenges in subsequent sections. The important thing to note is that gastroparesis can have repercussions even in the absence of gastrointestinal symptoms.

Very important

I'm not diabetic, so why would I have gastroparesis?

It's still a common misconception that gastroparesis is most often seen in diabetics. In actuality, idiopathic gastroparesis is the most common classification of the condition, making up about one-third of all cases. "Idiopathic" means that the cause is unknown. Post-viral gastroparesis is typically included in the idiopathic category, since it is difficult to confirm.

One of the things that makes gastroparesis so difficult to diagnose and manage, especially in idiopathic cases, is that it may be caused by a combination of factors, including genetics, environmental factors (such as surgery or a virus), and psychosocial factors.

Diabetes is the most common *known cause* of the condition. About 30 percent of gastroparesis cases are attributed to type 1 or type 2 diabetes. It's thought that erratic blood sugar damages the vagus nerve over time, impairing motility. Certain surgical procedures, particularly surgery on the abdomen, can result in post-surgical gastroparesis if the vagus nerve is damaged during the procedure. *gall bladde*
tomur on overies removed   hysteretomy
tubilagation

Other things that may cause delayed gastric emptying include acute eating disorders like anorexia nervosa, as well as underlying medical conditions such as hypothyroidism, mitochondrial disease, autoimmune conditions, collagen vascular disorders like scleroderma, and neurological conditions like Parkinson's disease.

Certain medications can also delay gastric emptying. These include:

- Narcotic pain medication   *Bi Polar meds Seroquel 500 Pm*
  Buspar 10 mg
  Am Pm

- Tricyclic antidepressants

- Anticholinergics (antispasmodics)

- Nicotine

- Progesterone

Progesterone? Does that include the birth control pill?

Some doctors believe that hormone-based birth control may contribute to delayed gastric emptying in some women. It's important to talk with your doctor about your use of birth control and to discuss whether or not you should discontinue hormone-based birth control for a period of time to see if it helps to alleviate symptoms.

It seems as if my gastroparesis symptoms get worse around my period. Is this common?

Because hormones can affect gastric emptying and overall GI motility, many women do notice that their symptoms ebb and flow along with their menstrual cycle. Once you identify this pattern, you may need to change your management strategy in the week or two prior to your period in order to sufficiently manage your symptoms.

Are people with gastroparesis more susceptible to colds and flus?

Whether it's due to poor nutrition, chronic stress, or something else, many GPers find that they are more susceptible to seasonal illnesses like colds and flus than they used to be. What's more, these acute illnesses often seem to linger longer than might otherwise be expected. Consistently addressing all areas of your gastroparesis management plan, including nutrition, lifestyle, and stress management, may help to strengthen your immune system and keep you healthier overall.

If you do get sick, keep in mind that liquid or chewable medication may be better tolerated than pills or tablets. Also note that certain medications can upset your stomach or exacerbate your gastroparesis symptoms, so you should talk with your doctor about alternatives that might be easier on the GI tract. Even after the illness has passed, you may notice an increase in GP symptoms and may need to alter your diet or other aspects of your management plan until things return to normal.

Does gastroparesis get worse over time?

If gastroparesis is caused by an underlying medical condition that is progressive in nature, then the dysmotility may also progress. But in the absence of an underlying condition, there is nothing about gastroparesis itself that suggests that the condition will get worse over time.

Some people do get worse, of course, but how much of that is related to the actual progression of the condition and how much is due to malnutrition and the extreme physical and mental stress that GP patients often endure is not clear. With proper medical management, adequate nutrition, and good self-care, it is not abnormal for patients to improve or even to get well over time.

If there's no cure for gastroparesis, does that mean I'll have it forever?

There is currently no medical cure for gastroparesis, but that doesn't mean that people never get better, nor does it mean that there will never be a cure. Medicine is evolving all the time. While very little is understood about functional gastrointestinal and motility disorders, research is ongoing. At this time, the prognosis for gastroparesis depends a great deal on its cause.

Delayed gastric emptying due to medication or an eating disorder is likely to resolve once the medication is removed or the patient begins taking in adequate nutrition. Gastroparesis resulting from an underlying condition, such as hypothyroidism, may resolve if the root problem is addressed. Diabetic gastroparesis tends to be long-lasting, though many diabetic gastroparetics are able to manage their symptoms via diet and lifestyle modifications. Post-viral gastroparesis is what I consider the "best case scenario" version of the condition, as it often resolves on its own within one to three years.

I've heard that gastroparesis can be fatal. Is this true?

Gastroparesis itself is not a fatal condition. People with gastroparesis *do* die, but not *because* their stomachs empty slowly. Typically, fatalities are due to complications that arise from severe malnutrition, infection, multiple system failures, or underlying causes such as mitochondrial disease.

This does not mean that gastroparesis is not a *life-altering* condition. It certainly is, and without adequate education, treatment, and self-care, it can be truly debilitating. Even with appropriate management, the condition can affect one's ability to work, socialize, or care for a family. The burden of living with gastroparesis and the impact it has on a patient's quality of life are terribly underestimated, but it is not a fatal condition in the vast majority of cases.

What's the most effective way to manage gastroparesis?

The first step in managing gastroparesis is realizing that it's a multi-faceted condition and must be approached from a variety of angles. In fact, it's the combination of medical treatments, complementary therapies, adequate nutrition, proper dietary modifications, a positive attitude, and supportive lifestyle practices that allow someone to actually *live well* with gastroparesis. None of these actions alone are likely to be as effective as when they are pursued collectively. Together they make up a comprehensive gastroparesis management plan.

Take another look at that list. The majority of what you can do to better manage gastroparesis falls under *self-care.* These are things *you* can do to improve your *own* outcomes. It's common to look to others—doctors, nutritionists, and experts of one kind or another—to make things better. I did just that for several years. But I can tell you from experience, things really start to improve when you take control of the situation, become your own advocate, and commit to practicing self-care.

Live Well Tip: Build a Dream Team

Surrounding yourself with a team of trusted experts makes medical management of gastroparesis much easier. I call this your Dream Team. It will take time and a good bit of effort to build this team. It's not something that happens immediately upon diagnosis, but once your Team is in place you should feel well supported in all aspects of your health and wellness.

The Team members will vary based on your current needs and may change over time. I've outlined the most common ones below.

Primary Care Provider

At the heart of your team should be a primary care or family doctor who acts as a liaison between your other specialists. This doctor should be familiar with your health history and all of your current medical concerns, and be able to provide you with referrals to specialists when necessary. While it's not necessary for a primary care provider to be an expert in gastroparesis (that's what your gastroenterologist is for, after all), you certainly want to feel as if he or she is as concerned about your well-being as you are. This is the Team member with whom you are likely to have the most contact, so choose wisely. Make sure he or she truly understands your needs and challenges, and is willing to work *with* you to address them.

Gastroenterologist/Motility Specialist

It's likely that your gastroparesis was diagnosed by a gastroenterologist, a doctor who treats disorders of the gastrointestinal tract. There are some gastroenterologists who specialize in motility disorders like gastroparesis. These doctors are called motility specialists. Having a doctor who specializes in, or is at least familiar with, gastroparesis will help to ensure that you have access to appropriate medical treatment. Depending on the severity of your symptoms, your health history, and whether you use medication to manage your symptoms, you may need to see your gastroenterologist frequently. Even if you don't need to see your gastroenterologist regularly, it is important to have one that you trust on your Team to address any changes in your symptoms or other concerns that may arise. You may need to meet with several doctors to find one who can best address your needs.

Mental Health Professional

While not necessary for everyone, a mental health provider (whether a licensed counselor, psychologist, or psychiatrist) can be a vital part of a successful management plan. Gastroparesis is not a mental disorder, but it can cause a significant amount of stress and anxiety. Having a trusted professional to help you work through these issues is mentally therapeutic and may actually help reduce your physical symptoms by reducing overall stress.

I especially recommend that you seek counseling if you have a history of disordered eating or if you begin to feel anxiety around eating due to gastroparesis.

Some mental health professionals specialize in treating patients who have chronic illness. For help finding a provider, visit www.nmha.org.

Nutrition Specialist

Most gastroparesis patients will benefit from a consultation with an experienced nutritional advisor, whether a registered dietitian, nutritionist, or a Certified Health Counselor. This is especially important if you have other dietary considerations, such as diabetes, celiac disease, multiple food allergies or intolerances, or if you plan to maintain a vegetarian or vegan diet.

Unfortunately, the majority of nutrition professionals have no experience dealing with gastroparesis and many are completely unfamiliar with the condition. Consulting an uninformed advisor can be a waste of your time and money, but worse still, uneducated recommendations can cause harm. So, just as with your gastroenterologist, you want to make sure that the nutrition professional you enlist for your Dream Team is knowledgeable and experienced in dealing with gastroparesis.

As far as I know, I am the only nutrition professional who currently specializes solely in gastroparesis management. However, your gastroenterologist may be able to recommend a local dietitian or nutritionist who is familiar with the condition.

Other Specialists

Depending on your medical history, you may need other specialists on your Dream Team. If new symptoms arise, you may require additional consultations or testing. Your primary care provider will help you determine which specialists you should be seeing.

Complementary Therapists

Your Team will also consist of any alternative or complementary health practitioners that you choose to work with, such as an acupuncturist or massage therapist. If they're not knowledgeable about gastroparesis, be sure that they are willing to learn. Be sure that all members of your Dream Team know about all treatments you are receiving, including complementary therapies. We'll talk more about complementary therapies for gastroparesis in the next section.

***

MEDICAL TREATMENT & COMPLEMENTARY THERAPY

Medical Treatment

The best interest of the patient is the only interest to be considered.

–Dr. W.J. Mayo

While much of what we can do to manage gastroparesis is based in self-care, the journey typically starts with a diagnosis from a doctor. Appropriate medical treatment can make a big difference in terms of alleviating symptoms and improving quality of life. What constitutes appropriate medical treatment may vary greatly from person to person depending on the severity of delayed gastric emptying, severity of symptoms, underlying conditions, and other health issues.

What kind of doctor treats gastroparesis?

Doctors who treat disorders of the gastrointestinal tract are called gastroenterologists. While there are gastroenterologists who specialize in motility disorders such as gastroparesis, they are few and far between. If you have access to one of these motility specialists, they are more likely to have the knowledge and means to provide you with a variety of treatment options, as well as more thorough diagnostic testing.

If there are no motility specialists in your area, you should find a general gastroenterologist who has experience with gastroparesis or is willing to work with you to learn more about the condition and the treatment options. Keep in mind that you may need to try several specialists before you find one who is a good fit for your needs.

Live Well Tip: How to Choose a Doctor

Deciding whether or not a doctor is a good fit for your needs can be difficult. Here are some things to consider as you make your decision:

- Does his/her office accept your insurance plan?

- Is his/her approach conservative or aggressive? Which do you prefer?

- Does he/she have experience with gastroparesis? If not, are they willing to learn about the condition and work *with* you as you learn to manage it?

- Does he/she express interest in and concern for your *quality of life*?

- Is his/her approach conventional or holistic? Which do you prefer?

- How available is he/she? How easy is it to reach him/her?

- How easy is it to get an appointment when you need one? Are you likely to see your practitioner or someone else in his/her office?

- Does he/she respond within a reasonable amount of time to phone messages? Can you reach them via email?

- Does he /she listen to your questions and take the time to answer them fully, in terms that you understand?

X • Does he/she ask your preferences and/or concerns about various treatment options?

• Are the office location and hours convenient for you?

X • Is the office staff friendly and helpful?

How can I find a motility specialist or doctor who is familiar with gastroparesis?

Finding the right doctor can be challenging. There are a few places you can start. The American Neurogastroenterology and Motility Society provides a list of doctors who specialize in motility disorders on their website: www.anms.org.

You can also visit the Enterra Therapy website at www.EnterraTherapy.com and click on "Find a Doctor." This will show you the surgeons in your area who implant the gastric neurostimulator. By contacting the surgeons' offices you'll likely be able to find out which gastroenterologists are referring patients for the gastric neurostimulator surgery. Those doctors will have experience treating patients with gastroparesis.

Finally, if you're in contact with other GPers in your area or are part of an online support group, ask about which doctors other people have seen and would recommend. Patient referrals are often the best resource.

I'm not sure my doctor takes me or my situation seriously. What should I do?

While many of us think of medical care as something best left to the experts, ultimately it's up to you to ensure that you are receiving appropriate and effective treatment. After all, you *hire* the people who provide it. If you're not satisfied with the treatment that your current doctor is willing or able to provide, then it's perfectly acceptable to move on. It doesn't mean that the doctor you're leaving isn't smart, capable, or a good doctor. It simply means that he or she isn't a good fit for *you* or your current situation. It's possible that your needs, and therefore the right doctor, may change over time. Don't be afraid to acknowledge when a fresh perspective is needed. Always be your own advocate.

Live Well Tip: Be an Expert Patient

Responsibility for your medical care does not lie solely with the doctor. Just as you expect him or her to take your situation seriously, you must do the same. You should strive to become a well-educated patient and a proactive participant in your own medical care. Here are some tips to help you do that:

- Bring a family member or trusted friend with you to all appointments and ask that they take notes. Sometimes it's hard to remember exactly what was said.

- Write down all of your questions and concerns in advance and bring them up early in the appointment.

- Be respectful of the doctor's time.

- Think about the questions your doctor may ask you and be prepared to answer them. Take some time prior to your appointment to think about your symptoms, how long you've had them, and what makes them better or worse.

- Bring any records or test results that you have from other doctors.

- Bring a list of all of prescription and over the counter medications, supplements, and vitamins you are currently taking, including dosage.

- Know which medications you have already tried for your symptoms and what the outcome was.

- Be specific. For example, rather than saying, "I can't eat much," outline what you eat in a typical day, including portion sizes.

- Ask questions when you don't understand something or you're not sure why your doctor is prescribing a certain medication.

- Ask for written instructions if you think it will help you understand or adhere to the doctor's recommendations.

- Always treat the doctor with respect, even if you don't agree with him or her.

Does everyone need medication to manage gastroparesis?

Typically, the first step in managing gastroparesis is to make dietary and lifestyle changes. For many people, these self-care techniques will sufficiently alleviate symptoms so that regular medication may not be necessary. Many GPers take medication only as needed to manage specific symptoms, such as nausea or pain.

If symptoms persist and/or affect other health issues, such as blood sugar management in diabetics, your doctor may recommend medication to speed up gastric emptying. Unfortunately the medications that are available to treat gastroparesis are not effective in all cases and it's likely that even with effective medication you'll need to carefully manage your diet and lifestyle in order to best manage symptoms.

What kinds of medication are available to treat gastroparesis?

Unfortunately, there aren't any medications that are universally effective for the treatment of gastroparesis. The drugs that are used typically have one of two purposes: either to increase the rate of gastric emptying or to manage symptoms like nausea, vomiting, or pain.

My doctor prescribed Reglan. What is it?   NO

Metoclopramide, better known by the brand name Reglan, is a prokinetic medication with a controversial reputation. It's recommended as first-line therapy by some practitioners and not at all by others. This medication is both a prokinetic, stimulating contractions of the stomach muscle to speed up gastric emptying, and an antiemetic, helping to alleviate nausea and vomiting.

Metoclopramide is known to cause tardive dyskinesia, a serious muscle disorder that is often permanent, especially at high doses and when used for an extended period of time. In 2009, the United States Food and Drug Administration (FDA) issued a black box warning for all metoclopramide-containing products. A black box warning means that medical studies indicate that the drug carries a significant risk of serious side effects, in this case tardive dyskinesia. Patients should inform their doctor *immediately* of any side effects experienced while taking this medication.

Other potential side effects of metoclopramide include: anxiety, restlessness, dizziness, drowsiness, and headache.

Are there any alternatives to Reglan?   NO

Aside from Reglan, erythromycin is the only FDA approved prokinetic medication. Erythromycin is an antibiotic that's used in very low doses to treat gastroparesis by increasing the contractions of the stomach. Its effectiveness appears to decrease over time, so it is typically recommended that patients cycle on and off the medication every few weeks or use it only during symptom flare-ups.

Potential side effects of erythromycin include: nausea, abdominal pain, and vomiting.

Domperidone, also known as Motilium, is similar to Reglan in that it is both a prokinetic and antiemetic drug. However, it does not carry the same risk of neurological side effects and is well tolerated by many patients who cannot tolerate or are not comfortable taking Reglan. FDA approval of domperidone is not being pursued in the U.S., but many patients are able to obtain it from reputable pharmacies in foreign countries, such as Canada and New Zealand, with a prescription from their doctor.

Potential side effects of domperidone include: constipation, dizziness, drowsiness, breast swelling, changes in menstrual cycle, and irregular heart rhythm.

Unfortunately, there isn't any one prokinetic medication that is effective for everyone with gastroparesis, and there is limited data comparing the efficacy of the various options. Talk with your doctor to determine which medication you should try first.

Is there anything new in the pipeline?

There are a number of drugs that are currently in development or are being reevaluated specifically for the treatment of gastroparesis. As awareness and research funding for motility disorders increases, additional treatment options will likely become available (see page 129).

One particular drug of note is TZP-102, which is currently in development by Tranzyme Pharma. As of 2011, the drug is in Phase II clinical trials. TZP-102 works differently from the other prokinetic medications currently available, targeting ghrelin receptors in the gut to stimulate emptying. In trials it has been shown to decrease nausea, early satiety, bloating, and upper abdominal pain in people with diabetic gastroparesis. TZP-102 was granted fast-track status by the FDA to expedite the approval process.

What if prokinetics don't work?

Often, prokinetic medications alone will not sufficiently reduce symptoms of gastroparesis. While we're waiting for more effective medications that actually treat the root problem, there are a variety of medications available to help with symptom management. Drugs that alleviate nausea and vomiting are called antiemetic medications. There are a variety of antiemetics available and, once again, it may be necessary to try several to find the one(s) that work best for you.

Common antiemetics used in the treatment of gastroparesis include Zofran, Tigan, Compazine, and Phenergan. Some of these can be used in combination or in rotation to enhance their effects. If you have trouble absorbing medication or experience frequent vomiting, you may want to ask your doctor for one that's available as a patch, suppository, or orally disintegrating tablet (ODT).

Potential side effects of antiemetic medications include: drowsiness, headache, and constipation.

Are there any non-prescription medications that help with nausea?

There are a number of over-the-counter medications that may help alleviate nausea. The one you're probably most familiar with is Pepto-Bismol. Another option, a favorite of mine and many of my clients, is a product called Nauzene. While these remedies are rarely effective for severe nausea or vomiting, they can be quite effective for relieving underlying queasiness.

Why did my doctor prescribe an antidepressant? I'm not depressed.

Some antidepressant medications, such as mirtazapine (Remeron), are used in low doses to treat gastroparesis. These medications have been shown to increase appetite, reduce feelings of fullness, and help alleviate pain in some patients. The major side effect of most of these drugs is drowsiness, which often decreases over time.

It's important to note that if your doctor recommends an antidepressant to treat gastroparesis, he or she is not saying that you are depressed or that your symptoms are in your head. These medications work on the neurotransmitters in the gut which help to regulate digestion and transfer messages from the stomach to the brain and vice versa, thus decreasing symptoms.

How can I manage pain?

Pain can be one of the most difficult gastroparesis symptoms to manage. For cases of mild pain, relaxation exercises or gentle physical activity may be quite helpful. Heat can be an effective treatment for the abdominal and chest pain associated with gastroparesis. I highly recommend that you invest in a good heating pad or hot/cold pack. Heat draws blood into the organs, helping them work more effectively. Heat will also help to relax and alleviate any cramping or spasms that you might experience within the GI tract.

For some people who have gastroparesis, the pain can be severe and disabling. If over-the-counter medications like Tylenol or ibuprofen do not provide adequate relief, there are a variety of medications that can be prescribed by a doctor.

Serotonin-norepinephrine reuptake inhibitor (SNRI) antidepressants, such as Cymbalta, have been shown to decrease the pain associated with functional GI and motility disorders.

Neurontin and Lyrica, both of which have been studied primarily in diabetic gastroparesis, may also help alleviate pain by dulling the nerves in the gut.

The least desirable option for managing gastroparesis-related pain is narcotic pain medication such as hydrocodone and oxycodone. These drugs have been shown to delay motility throughout the entire gastrointestinal tract. So while they help to alleviate pain, they may actually exacerbate other gastroparesis symptoms and/or cause constipation.

Tramadol is a prescription pain medication that is not technically a narcotic and, in low doses, does not seem to delay gastric emptying. It can be habit-forming, however, so it's not ideal for long-term use.

Are over-the-counter antacids GP-friendly?

Many over-the-counter antacids, such as Maalox, contain aluminum hydroxide, which is known to delay gastric emptying. Tums and Rolaids are a better choice. There are also a number of herbal remedies available for the treatment of acid reflux (see page 32).

Does chewing gum help with acid reflux?

Several recent studies have shown that chewing gum can help alleviate the symptoms of acid reflux by forcing fluids back into the stomach and neutralizing acids that cause heartburn. Chewing gum for about an hour after meals may also help facilitate gastric emptying by increasing the production of digestive juices.

Keep in mind that chewing gum causes you to swallow more air, which may exacerbate bloating and belching. The artificial sweeteners found in most sugar-free gums can also exacerbate stomach pain and/or bloating in some people.

Does everyone with gastroparesis need acid reflux mediation?

In many cases, people with gastroparesis are initially diagnosed with acid reflux or GERD (gastroesophageal reflux disease) and put on acid suppressing medication, commonly a proton pump inhibitor (PPI) like Nexium, Prevacid, Aciphex, or Prilosec. When further testing eventually reveals gastroparesis, many people are never taken off of the acid suppressing drugs or reevaluated to confirm the initial GERD diagnosis.

Not everyone who has gastroparesis has acid reflux. In general, we need some acid in our stomach in order to break down and digest food. For many people with gastroparesis, the problem is not that there is too much acid being produced; it's that the acid that is present refluxes into the esophagus once the stomach gets full. Suppressing the production of acid may actually cause food to remain in the stomach longer, since the stomach contents must reach a certain level of acidity before emptying begins. In fact, recent studies have found that PPIs can delay gastric emptying in healthy volunteers.

There are, of course, many cases in which these medications are appropriate and necessary: if acid damage is found in the stomach or esophagus, for example, or severe acid reflux is documented via a 24-hour pH study or wireless capsule. Always talk with your doctor before starting or stopping any medication.

Are Botox injections effective for the treatment of gastroparesis?

There isn't a great deal of scientific evidence that Botox injections are effective for the treatment of gastroparesis, but about half of the patients who receive the procedure report reduced symptoms. Some studies have found similar results with an injection of saline, suggesting either a placebo effect or a potential therapeutic benefit from the injection itself.

The botulinum toxin (Botox), which is injected during an upper endoscopy, causes the pylorus to relax, thereby allowing food to empty from the stomach into the small intestine more quickly with the help of gravity. The effects of Botox are temporary, typically lasting about two to six months on average. Repeat injections can be given, though there is no guarantee that they will continue to be effective.

Personally, I've had the procedure done twice. The first time, I noticed a significant reduction in my symptoms, which lasted for about eight weeks. After the results wore off, I received another injection. Unfortunately I didn't notice any improvement that time.

Not all gastroenterologists offer Botox treatment and insurance coverage for the procedure varies. Given the temporary effects and approximately fifty-fifty chance of success, it's a personal decision as to whether or not it's worth trying.

What is gastric electrical stimulation?

Gastric electrical stimulation is a relatively new treatment option for patients with drug-refractory nausea and vomiting due to gastroparesis. It involves the implantation of a device called a gastric neurostimulator, which is about the size of a pocket watch, under the skin in the abdomen. Leads are attached to both the device and the stomach muscle and transfer electric pulses every few seconds. How the device actually works isn't completely understood, but it's thought to affect the nerves that register sensations within the stomach.

Though it is not a cure for gastroparesis and does not typically lead to an improvement in gastric emptying time, gastric electrical stimulation does alleviate nausea and vomiting in the majority of recipients. Several studies have found that patients also report a better quality of life and spend less time in the hospital following placement of the device.

Enterra Therapy was approved by the FDA in 2000 as a Humanitarian Use Device and should therefore be covered by insurance providers. Patients who are dependent on narcotic drugs, currently pregnant, or unable to undergo surgery are typically not considered good candidates for the procedure.

For more information, or to find a doctor in your area who specializes in gastric electrical stimulation, visit www.EnterraTherapy.com.

Is the gastric neurostimulator the same as the gastric pacemaker?

The gastric neurostimulator is often called a gastric pacemaker. While most people mean the same thing by both terms, "pacemaker" is actually a misnomer. The device doesn't pace the stomach muscle in the way that a heart pacemaker paces the heart muscle. You may also hear it called a gastric stimulator, gastric pacer, or the Enterra device. The treatment itself may be referred to as either Enterra Therapy or gastric electrical stimulation (GES—not to be confused with a gastric emptying study!).

Think of it this way: Enterra is the brand name of the gastric neurostimulator, which is implanted for gastric electrical stimulation.

How do I know if the gastric neurostimulator is right for me?

The gastric neurostimulator isn't appropriate for everyone. You must be able to undergo and recover from surgery, including general anesthesia. While the treatment is primarily indicated for symptoms due to idiopathic and diabetic gastroparesis, some medical centers only offer the procedure to diabetic patients, since the response is more predictable among this group. In addition, many doctors won't implant the device in people who are dependent on narcotic pain medicine, since narcotics slow transit throughout the gastrointestinal tract.

Only your doctor can help you to determine whether or not you're a good candidate for the procedure. I'd also recommend asking to meet with the Enterra representative and the surgeon who will potentially perform your surgery to ensure that you're able to get all of your questions answered. Proper preparation will likely lead to a better outcome.

My Experience with the Gastric Neurostimulator

I had my first gastric neurostimulator implanted in September 2009 at the Mayo Clinic in Rochester, Minnesota. Unfortunately, that one malfunctioned, so I had the entire system replaced on January 19, 2010. It's been nearly two years since then and I can honestly say that the treatment has dramatically improved my quality of life.

Enterra Therapy has not cured me of gastroparesis or even eliminated my symptoms. But it has significantly reduced both the severity and frequency of my most debilitating symptom: nausea. Before I had the gastric neurostimulator implanted, the nausea was unrelenting. My diet was extremely limited and I wasn't able to sleep more than two or three hours each night. The weight loss, lack of nutrition, and sleep deprivation took as much of a toll on my health and quality of life as the gastroparesis itself.

Thanks to the gastric neurostimulator, I'm now nausea-free most of the time so long as I follow the rest of my comprehensive management plan. Depending on the ebb and flow of my symptoms, I only have difficulty sleeping once or twice per month—a big improvement from four to five times per week! I've also been able to gain and maintain ten pounds since the second device was implanted. In addition to allowing me to increase the variety and nutrition in my everyday diet, the treatment has given me some extra leeway with my dietary choices on special occasions, such as birthday and holidays.

I still have to manage my symptoms with careful dietary choices, proper nutrition, lots of physical activity, stress management, and Zofran, on occasion, but the gastric neurostimulator is an integral part of my management plan. Without it, those other things wouldn't work nearly as well. While Enterra Therapy isn't a cure for gastroparesis, it's the best symptom management tool I've found and it has changed my life.

Will I need a feeding tube?

In a small minority of GP cases, somewhere around 15 percent, artificial nutrition via feeding tubes or intravenous therapy (IV) may be necessary in order to prevent malnutrition, treat dehydration, stabilize blood sugar, and/or deliver medication. There are two kinds of artificial nutrition: enteral and parenteral. Both methods are usually temporary.

Enteral nutrition is commonly referred to as tube feeding. A jejunostomy tube, or "J tube," is placed into the small intestine, bypassing the stomach. This may be necessary in cases of extreme malnutrition and/or dehydration, or in patients with diabetic gastroparesis if the delayed emptying prevents medication necessary for maintaining blood sugar from entering the bloodstream. A gastrostomy tube, or "G tube," may also be surgically placed through the skin on the abdomen directly into the stomach to drain or vent the stomach.

Total parenteral nutrition is delivered intravenously, bypassing the digestive tract entirely. Nutrients are given through a catheter which goes directly into the bloodstream. Also called TPN, this treatment is used only in the most severe cases.

Again, most gastroparesis patients will never require artificial nutrition.

What about the gastric sleeve or gastric band?

Surgery to bypass, remove, or in some other way alter the stomach is rarely used to treat gastroparesis. Few studies have been done to determine the efficacy of these surgeries, but so far the results have been mixed. While some patients have reported improvement of symptoms, in some cases gastroparesis has been a *result* of these procedures. Currently, surgical interventions such as the gastric band, gastric sleeve, or gastric bypass are considered a last resort and are very rarely indicated.

Complementary Therapy

The part can never be well unless the whole is well.

–Plato

Complementary treatments are therapies and remedies that don't typically fall within the realm of conventional medicine. They are often holistic in nature, targeting both physical and emotional aspects of gastroparesis. These treatments can be quite effective for managing symptoms such as pain, nausea, vomiting, insomnia, and/or anxiety. They're called complementary because they are used *in conjunction with* conventional medicine and other treatment strategies to enhance effects and benefits overall. Some people who are refractory to medical treatment find relief with complementary treatment.

Are there any natural supplements or herbal remedies that can improve gastric emptying?

There are a handful of non-pharmaceutical remedies that can help to facilitate gastric emptying. These include: ginger, Iberogast, and bitters.

You're probably familiar with ginger as an effective and time-tested remedy for an upset stomach. In addition to alleviating nausea, ginger has been found to speed up gastric emptying in healthy volunteers. Ginger is available in a variety of forms, from tea to capsules to gum. Ingesting 1,200 mg prior to meals may help to enhance digestion and reduce symptoms.

potassium?

While most Americans are unfamiliar with Iberogast this liquid herbal formula has been used for decades in Europe to alleviate symptoms of dyspepsia such as heartburn and bloating. Studies have shown that it may also speed up gastric emptying. Iberogast has a good safety record with few reported side effects.

Bitters are similar to Iberogast and enhance digestion by increasing gastric juices and stimulating the production of enzymes. The smooth muscle of the stomach is stimulated by the bitter reflex, so ingesting bitters may lead to an increase in gastric motility. Bitters also cause the esophageal sphincter to contract, preventing the reflux of stomach contents into the esophagus.

How about remedies to alleviate the symptoms of gastroparesis?

Peppermint oil has been found to reduce nausea, abdominal pain, bloating, and gas in people with functional gastrointestinal disorders. While peppermint oil capsules are available, many GPers find peppermint tea a more effective and immediate remedy for symptoms. Note that if you have acid reflux, peppermint tea may exacerbate the condition by relaxing the lower esophageal sphincter (LES).

Other potentially effective remedies for nausea include fennel and chamomile tea.

A safe, effective, and inexpensive remedy for the burning and reflux that many GPers experience is deglycerized licorice (DGL). Chewing DGL tablets, which can be used in conjunction with over-the-counter and prescription GERD medication, coats and soothes the stomach and esophagus.

Another heartburn remedy that can also alleviate constipation and help to heal the GI tract is aloe vera juice. There are a number of aloe vera juices on the market, and some of them taste better than others. I've found Aloe Life Cherry Berry to be the most pleasant in terms of flavor.

Are digestive enzymes helpful for gastroparesis?

Our bodies naturally produce over twenty kinds of digestive enzymes, each of which acts on a specific type of food. The role of these enzymes, found in our saliva, stomach, pancreas, and small intestine, is to help break down the food we eat so that the body can absorb the nutrients.

Most people with healthy digestive tracts naturally produce an adequate amount of enzymes, and raw foods contain their own enzymes, so digestive enzyme supplements generally aren't necessary. However, people with impaired digestion, especially those of us with gastroparesis who cannot eat a variety of fresh, raw foods, may notice a reduction in bloating, belching, and heartburn with the use of supplemental enzymes. These supplements may also help with nutrient absorption in some cases.

There are a dizzying number of digestive enzyme supplements on the market. A complete enzyme formula will contain amylase to break down carbohydrates, lipase to break down fats, protease to break down protein, cellulase to break down fiber, and lactase to break down dairy products.

Some of the more potent formulas may actually exacerbate digestive discomfort, so it's always a good idea to start with less than the recommended amount and work up gradually. If you follow a vegetarian diet, avoid products containing pancreatin, since it's derived from animal enzymes. Experimentation may be necessary to find which formula, if any, helps to reduce your symptoms. One simple place to start is with a chewable papaya enzyme. These are readily available and inexpensive.

Should people with gastroparesis take probiotics?

Our large intestine is naturally full of bacteria—some that are helpful and some that may be harmful if they become too numerous. When the "bad" bacteria outnumber the "good," effects can include bloating, gas, cramping and bowel changes. Probiotic supplements provide extra good bacteria, which may help to alleviate those symptoms and restore balance in the colon.

Like digestive enzymes, there are many probiotic formulas available. These products contain a wide variety of bacteria strains, some of which are more helpful than others. Bacillus coagulans (BC-30) and Lactobacillus GG have been found to be particularly effective for relieving GI symptoms.

While probiotics are not likely to improve gastroparesis directly, they may improve lower gastrointestinal symptoms such as bloating, gas, pain, and bowel irregularity.

Is there anything I should know before I try these kinds of supplements?

Not all herbal remedies or supplements are appropriate for everyone. Most are not regulated by the FDA. Before you start taking anything (even herbal or "natural" products), make sure to educate yourself about the potential risks and interactions with medications or other supplements. Always tell your doctor and other practitioners about *all* products that you're taking, including herbal and dietary supplements. Also, keep in mind that not all of these remedies will work equally well for everyone. You may need to try a variety of supplements to find the exact formulas that work best for you.

Live Well Tip: Learn to Love Ginger

Take a peek in my fridge, purse or pantry, and you'll find some form of ginger in each one. I'm a big fan of natural remedies that actually work and not only is ginger a time-tested treatment for nausea and digestive discomfort, it's also been found to speed gastric emptying. If it's not currently part of your management plan, I encourage you to give it a try. There are tons of ginger products available, but here's a rundown of my favorites.

Ginger Tea

Tea—Perfect for late night (or middle-of-the-night) bouts of nausea, ginger tea can be made from fresh ginger or from purchased tea bags. Try drinking a cup about 30 minutes before meals to stimulate gastric juices or after meals to aid digestion. (See the recipe on page 220)

Ginger Ale

Soda—There's a reason your mom gave you ginger ale when you had an upset stomach—it works! If you find that the carbonation exacerbates bloating or belching, let the soda sit open for a while before drinking. Some brands don't actually contain ginger, so check the ingredient label. Also, avoid high-fructose corn syrup and artificial sweeteners whenever possible. My favorite ginger ale is from Zevia; it is made with stevia, an herbal sweetener.

Stevia

Syrup—Ginger syrup (also called tonic) is usually a mixture of ginger extract and honey. It can be taken directly off the spoon (like cough syrup), stirred into hot water, mixed with soda water, or even added to smoothies or juice.

 Capsules—If you tolerate capsules, taking 1,200 mg two to three times a day is one of the easiest ways to reap the benefits of ginger. If you experience ginger-flavored burps when taking capsules during the day, try taking a dose before bed instead to help alleviate middle-of-the-night nausea.

Crystallized/Candied Ginger—These chewy, bite-size pieces of preserved ginger are sweet, spicy, and very effective for alleviating nausea. Some find crystallized ginger too fibrous and/or spicy.

Ginger Candies—Less intense and certainly more kid-friendly than crystallized ginger, ginger candies come in both hard and soft varieties. They're great to keep in your purse or pocket while you're out and about, especially while traveling. For kids with GP, sucking on ginger candies can be a discreet way to manage nausea during the school day. My favorites are Gin-Gins hard candy and Ginger Chews from The Ginger People.

Cookies—I don't recommend eating ginger cookies as a primary strategy for managing symptoms, but they can help to settle the stomach. I prefer homemade (see the recipe on page 230), but you can find low-fat ginger snaps in the grocery store. Just make sure ginger is actually listed as an ingredient!

Is acupuncture helpful for gastroparesis?

Acupuncture is the most widely researched of all complementary therapies. It's been shown to reduce nausea, vomiting, and pain, as well as anxiety, fatigue, depression, and insomnia.

Acupuncture involves inserting thin, sterile needles into the body along energy pathways called meridians. Treatments are generally not painful and can actually be quite relaxing.

You'll likely need several sessions before you notice significant results. However, if you don't notice any benefit after four to six sessions, either the treatment or the practitioner may not be right for you. The practitioner is very important, because the way in which they perform the treatment, as well as their level of experience, can make a difference in the results you experience. Just as not every doctor is a good fit for you, neither will every complementary practitioner be.

To find a qualified acupuncturist, visit www.medicalacupuncture.org (all of the members are licensed physicians) or www.nccaom.org.

Electroacupuncture is performed similarly to traditional acupuncture, except once the needles are inserted they are connected to small electrodes which periodically deliver electrical pulses to enhance the effect. Few studies have been done to evaluate the efficacy of electroacupuncture.

Are there any other treatments that are effective for alleviating symptoms?

While most people think of hypnosis as affecting the mind, it can also have significant effects on the body, including the GI tract. Hypnotherapy is a technique that combines guided relaxation and focused attention to induce a heightened state of awareness, which enables changes in perception and the potential to control bodily functions that are usually involuntary. Gut-directed hypnotherapy is a special form of hypnosis that has been shown to relieve symptoms associated with functional gastrointestinal disorders.

To find a qualified hypnotherapist, visit www.aaph.org.

Massage therapy may lower levels of stress hormones and alleviate anxiety, both of which can contribute to a worsening of gastroparesis symptoms. It is also thought that massage improves the regulation of the autonomic nervous system, which plays an important role in digestion. Abdominal massage, in particular, may be especially beneficial for patients with gastroparesis, especially those struggling with constipation.

To find a qualified massage therapist, visit www.amtamassage.org.

Craniosacral therapy (CST) is a hands-on method of enhancing the craniosacral system, which comprises the membranes and fluid that surround and protect the brain and spinal cord. According to CST practitioners, these tissues control the development and performance of the central nervous system. Practitioners use a soft touch to release restrictions in the body's fascia and craniosacral system in order to improve the functioning of the central nervous system. This may be helpful for gastroparesis patients, especially those who experienced a physical or mental trauma prior to the onset of symptoms.

To find a qualified therapist, visit www.Upledger.com or www.MilneInstitute.com.

Are these treatments covered by health insurance plans?

Acupuncture, electroacupuncture, and massage therapy treatments are covered by some insurance plans, but not by others. Hypnotherapy and craniosacral therapy are typically not covered by insurance, though you should check with your insurance company to be sure.

Live Well Tip: Choosing Complementary Therapy Practitioners

When considering complementary therapies, it's important to find a well-qualified, knowledgeable practitioner with whom you feel comfortable. The skill and background of the practitioner, as well as whether or not you are at ease during the treatments, often plays a role in the outcome of therapy. Here are a few tips when choosing a practitioner:

- Talk with your doctor(s) and let them know that you're considering complementary therapies. Whether or not they are able to recommend a practitioner, they need to be aware of all treatments you are receiving. For tips about talking with your health care providers about complementary medicine, visit http://nccam.nih.gov/timetotalk/.

- Call or visit the website of the professional organization for the treatment you are considering. Most offer a directory of qualified practitioners or will be able to instruct you on where to find such a list.

- Tell family, friends, and acquaintances about your search for a practitioner. You'd be surprised how many will chime in with recommendations.

- Gather basic information about the practitioners you are considering, such as their education, experience, cost, and insurance options, and interview them in person or by telephone. You may want to ask about their specific experience with gastroparesis. Having no experience shouldn't necessarily rule out a given practitioner, but you want to gauge their willingness to learn about your condition and the way in which they will approach something they may know little about.

- Evaluate your practitioner after the initial visit and decide if the practitioner is right for you.

Are there any complementary therapies I can do on my own?

Though treatment performed by a qualified professional may be the most effective, self-care versions of these therapies are extremely valuable since you can do them more frequently and whenever you experience acute symptoms.

Acupressure is similar to acupuncture in that specific points along energy meridians are stimulated to relieve certain symptoms. In acupressure, the points are stimulated with touch rather than needles. This is something you can learn to do on your own, anywhere and at any time. To alleviate nausea, for example, find the point on the inside of your wrist that is about three finger lengths down and between the two major tendons. Massage in gentle circles for up to two minutes. Avoid pressing too hard; doing so can occasionally make nausea worse. You can also purchase acupressure wristbands that apply continuous pressure to this point. They are sold over the counter in most drug stores.

Abdominal massage is also easy to learn and perform on yourself. Practice by lying down with your abdominal muscles relaxed. Starting at your belly button, use gentle pressure to massage the abdomen in a clockwise direction, slowly moving outward. It might be helpful to ask a qualified practitioner to demonstrate the technique for you. Do not massage your abdomen if you have cancer, an ulcer, a heart condition, high blood pressure, or if you are pregnant.

Self-hypnosis or guided imagery can help alleviate a variety of physical symptoms as well as anxiety and insomnia. It's easily practiced at home with a CD or DVD, though you may need to experiment to find the one that best suits you.

Dietary Modifications

When it comes to diet, one size definitely doesn't fit all.

–Christiane Northrup, M.D.

Diet tends to be the subject that those of us with gastroparesis spend the most time and energy agonizing over. Understandably so. After all, symptoms are usually related to eating and a great deal of emphasis is put on dietary modification for symptom management. Unfortunately, guidance and information about how to actually make appropriate dietary changes is often lacking. In addition, no studies have been conducted to figure out the best diet for managing gastroparesis symptoms, so the recommendations are based primarily on the science of healthy digestion.

Based on my work with clients and my own experience, I've come up with ten guidelines for eating for gastroparesis:

- Eat smaller meals.

- Eat *less* fiber.

- Eat *less* fat.

- Maximize the nutrition in each bite and sip.

- Avoid food with indigestible parts.

- Add nutrient-dense soft foods and liquids. ✶ avacado

- Keep a food journal.

- Chew thoroughly. ✶

- Eat slowly and in a relaxed environment.

- Do what works *for you.*

What do you mean do what works for me? Aren't there specific rules I need to follow?

What works for one person with gastroparesis won't always work for the next. That's because gastroparesis isn't one condition with one presentation. While the diagnosis is the same, gastric emptying times can range from nearly normal to extremely delayed. Likewise, the type and severity of symptoms, as well as the underlying cause, varies from person to person. For these reasons, there's no such thing as a one-size-fits-all diet for gastroparesis management. However the guidelines above will help you figure out what works best for *you.*

Live Well Tip: Understanding "Gastroparesis-friendly"

You'll see the term *gastroparesis-friendly* or *GP-friendly* used throughout this book in reference to foods and recipes. When I describe something as GP-friendly, I'm indicating that:

- It doesn't contain anything that is known to cause bezoars or blockages. No nuts, seeds, skins, hulls, peels, dried fruit, raw vegetables, etc.

- It follows the general gastroparesis diet guidelines, meaning that it's relatively low in fat, low in fiber, and easy to digest.

- It's likely to be well tolerated by many GPers.

Anything that meets these criteria is unlikely to cause any serious problems (i.e., it's not going to make the gastroparesis worse overall). However, there are things that I deem

"GP-friendly" that I personally don't tolerate very well and there are likely to be some that you won't tolerate very well either. So while I can tell you what tends to be GP-friendly, careful and consistent experimentation is really the only way to know for sure what is <*your name here*>-friendly.

Here's a quick rundown of things to keep in mind as you build a GP-friendly diet:

- As part of a comprehensive management plan, dietary modifications can be a very effective tool for managing the symptoms of gastroparesis.

- The gastroparesis-friendly diet is not a treatment for the condition itself. Your stomach may certainly begin to function properly again over time, but not because you removed fat and/or fiber from your diet.

- Eating a food or a meal that is not "gastroparesis-friendly" may exacerbate symptoms in the short term because the food will digest more slowly, but it will not make the condition worse overall.*

- For most people, there is a point at which continuing to restrict the diet will not further alleviate symptoms. An overly restricted diet may lead to malnutrition and other consequent health issues.

The exception is in cases of bezoar formation (see page 48). To be on the safe side, people with gastroparesis should avoid the foods most associated with bezoar formation, including apple peels, berries, broccoli, Brussels sprouts, coconuts, corn, green beans, figs, oranges, persimmons, potato peels, sauerkraut, and tomato skins. Also use caution with nuts, seeds, and beans/ legumes.

Will following a GP-friendly diet cure my gastroparesis?

A gastroparesis-friendly diet is a tool for managing symptoms. It's not a treatment for dysmotility or a cure for gastroparesis itself. While gastroparesis can get better or even completely resolve over time, it's not the result of following a GP-friendly diet.

So a gastroparesis-friendly diet won't speed up my emptying time?

I often hear people say that eating less fat or less fiber will speed up gastric emptying. This isn't true. A gastroparesis-friendly diet won't *speed up* gastric emptying. It will just prevent the stomach from emptying more slowly.

When you had your gastric emptying scan, the meal that you were given was most likely small, low-fat and low-fiber. It was basically a gastroparesis-friendly meal. You emptied that GP-friendly meal slowly. That's why you were diagnosed with delayed gastric emptying. Your "baseline" emptying rate is slow, and following a GP-friendly diet will not eliminate or shorten that existing delay.

Then what's the point of the gastroparesis-friendly diet?

Dietary modifications are an essential part of a comprehensive gastroparesis management plan. While it's not a cure-all, following a gastroparesis-friendly diet can *significantly* reduce symptoms. Foods that are higher in fat and/or fiber take longer to empty from the stomach than foods lower in fat and fiber. This is true for everybody, even people without gastroparesis. So when we choose GP-friendly foods, it allows the stomach to empty as quickly as possible given the existing delay, and therefore helps to alleviate symptoms.

If I still don't feel well, should I continue cutting foods out of my diet?

Unfortunately, modifying the diet will not completely eliminate symptoms for most people with gastroparesis. Dietary changes are a symptom-management tool, and there comes a point at which further restriction of your diet will not provide additional benefit in terms of reducing symptoms. Regardless of how little fat or fiber you eat, your stomach will still empty slowly.

When you continue to restrict your diet past the point of symptom management benefit, you risk malnutrition. This can make both digestion and overall health worse, as the body needs adequate nourishment in order to function properly. So, while dietary modification is an important part of a gastroparesis management plan, it's only *one* part and we cannot focus solely on diet with the expectation that it will alleviate all of our symptoms.

If I eat something that's not gastroparesis-friendly once in a while, will it make my gastroparesis worse overall?

Eating food that is not considered gastroparesis-friendly will not make the condition worse overall, nor will it do any damage to your stomach. Certainly you may feel worse in the short term, since non-GP-friendly foods take longer to empty and are therefore more likely to exacerbate symptoms, but you don't need to worry about doing yourself any long-term harm.

Are there any foods that I definitely should not eat?

To be on the safe side, you should avoid foods that have indigestible parts or foods that are hard to chew completely. These can further delay gastric emptying and may in some cases lead to bezoars. In general, it's best to steer clear of raw vegetables; whole nuts and seeds; any skins, peels, or hulls; all legumes and dried beans; dried fruit; shredded coconut; berries, including cherries and grapes; broccoli; and corn (including popcorn).

Can I eat these foods if I puree them?

Part of the stomach's job is to grind food into particles small enough to be emptied into the small intestine, about 1-2 mm. Pureeing your food helps the stomach do this more quickly, especially in cases where the muscles aren't contracting properly. If you choose to experiment with foods like beans, berries, or harder-to-digest veggies, pureeing them is a good place to start.

For example, while chickpeas are not gastroparesis-friendly, many GPers do fine with small amounts of very smooth hummus (1-2 tablespoons). Keep in mind that pureeing foods doesn't change the fiber content; it simply makes them easier for the stomach to grind and empty.

What is a bezoar, and should I be worried about getting one?

Bezoars are hardened masses of undigested food. They can block the outlet of the stomach, causing a severe exacerbation of symptoms such as vomiting and fullness. Only about 20 percent of all GPers will ever get a bezoar. Once you've had one, however, you're more prone to getting another. Foods specifically associated with bezoar formation are apples, berries, broccoli, Brussels sprouts, coconuts, corn, green beans, figs, oranges, persimmons, potato peels, and sauerkraut. Fiber supplements such as Metamucil, Perdiem, Benefiber, Fibercon, and Citrucel can also contribute to the formation of bezoars.

Why does eating smaller meals help with gastroparesis, and how small do my meals need to be?

Most of us, if given any direction at all upon diagnosis, were told to eat six or more small meals per day rather than three regular-sized meals. That's because volume is the largest determinant of gastric emptying time. Reducing the size of a meal helps to decrease the amount of time it takes for the stomach to empty it. For those of us with gastroparesis, an appropriate meal size is approximately one-third to one-half the size of a "normal" meal, or about one to one and a half cups of foods.

How many times a day should I eat?

Depending on how many hours you're awake and how much you can comfortably eat at each meal, you may need to eat anywhere between five and eight meals per day. To figure out the best meal pattern for you, check out the experimentation tips on page 60.

That's a lot of meals to prepare. Wouldn't it be easier just to snack all day instead?

While it may be easier to simply snack or "graze" all day long, it's doesn't lead to the best symptom management. Snack foods, especially those that are low in fat and fiber, tend to be empty foods—they take up space without providing much in the way of nutrition. You're likely to get too many carbohydrates and too much sugar, but too little protein and healthy fat.

Grazing can also lead to overeating. In fact, while you might only be having a couple of bites at a time, those bites add up and may you leave you feeling more full and symptomatic than if you ate several small meals.

Defined mealtimes also facilitate better digestion. When you're constantly eating, you're continuously adding more food to the stomach, possibly before it's even started digesting your last snack. Think of it this way: if you were cooking a big pot of beans and you kept adding more uncooked beans, your pot would never be fully cooked. Give your stomach some time to work before you give it more work to do.

So I have to prepare six or more meals every day?

While eating six well-balanced mini-meals is ideal, it's not always realistic. A good goal is to aim for *at least* three mini-meals: breakfast, lunch and dinner. At these times, make your plate look like a "normal" meal, which means including more than one food group, only in smaller portions. The other three to four mini-meals can be well-balanced snacks.

If you work outside the home or are otherwise away from home for most of the day, you may need to prepare your meals ahead of time. Consider making and freezing individual portions of purees, soups, and smoothies. You can also prepackage individual servings of crackers and cereal, and/or bake up several potatoes and sweet potatoes in advance. You can even make and freeze individual portions of cooked hot cereal and white rice. Having these "grab and go" staples on hand will make it much easier to adhere to a balanced GP-friendly diet throughout the day.

Live Well Tip: Grab & Go GP-Friendly Meals

Keep these portable staples on hand and you'll always have a well-balanced, GP-friendly meal or snack that you can grab on the run.

No Refrigeration Necessary

? • Orgain (no refrigeration needed; pour over ice when ready to drink)

- MacroBars or other protein bars

- Organic pureed vegetable soups, such as Imagine Foods brand

- Individual packets of instant Cream of Wheat (just add hot water, a small sliced or mashed banana and a tablespoon of creamy nut butter for a well-balanced meal)

- English muffins or low-fat graham crackers (spread with nut butter)

- Low-fiber crackers (eat with cheese or spread with nut butter)

- Individual serving size packets of creamy peanut butter or smooth almond butter

- Individual servings of applesauce, baby food fruits, canned peaches, or canned pears (stir into low-fat cottage cheese, Greek yogurt or non-dairy yogurt)

- Ripe bananas

- Microwavable white potatoes and/or sweet potatoes

Perishable

- Frozen homemade smoothies

- Homemade soups

- Individual servings of Greek yogurt

- Individual servings of cottage cheese

- Homemade fruit or vegetable purees

- Hard-boiled eggs

- Mini Babybel Light cheese

Why do I need to limit fiber?

Foods that are high in fiber take longer to empty from the stomach than lower-fiber foods. That's true for everyone, whether they have gastroparesis or not. Fiber is simply more difficult to break down and therefore requires more time for digestion. Decreasing the total amount of fiber in your diet and avoiding high-fiber foods will allow your meals to empty from the stomach as quickly as possible (given your existing delay), thereby lessening the symptoms of gastroparesis.

What exactly does "low fiber" mean? How low?

Low fiber does not mean no fiber. We all need some fiber in our diets in order to regulate bowel movements and cleanse the gastrointestinal tract, among other things. It's important to find a balance between minimizing symptoms and obtaining an adequate amount of fiber for good health. Even if you eliminated *all* fiber from the diet, it wouldn't normalize your gastric emptying. The specific amount of fiber tolerated by GPers varies from person to person, but it's usually between 10 and 15 grams per day.

How do I reduce fiber in a healthy way?

There are two ways to go about reducing fiber in the diet. The first is to completely eliminate foods like whole grains, fruits, and vegetables. While this is probably the most common approach, it's not the one I recommend. This typically leaves mostly processed, nutritionally poor foods that do little more than take up space in your stomach.

The second approach, the one I recommend, is to incorporate small portions of GP-friendly versions of higher-fiber foods, like cooked vegetables, pureed soups, fruit smoothies, fresh juices, hot cereals, and smooth nut butters, and fill in the gaps with lower-fiber choices like white potatoes, rice, pasta, and bread.

How do I know if I'm eating too little fiber? How can I safely add more?

In general, most gastroparesis patients do best with a maximum of about 15 grams of fiber per day, which is actually right around the average intake for all Americans. If you're getting much less than 15 grams per day, you can experiment by slowly replacing some of the GP-friendly "empty" foods in your diet—such as white rice, white pasta, white crackers, sugary cereals, white bread—with well-cooked and/or pureed GP-friendly fruits and veggies, like sweet potatoes, carrots, turnips, parsnips, pumpkin, beets, bananas, applesauce, canned pears, and canned peaches. Choose just one food to replace each week until your symptoms increase or you reach about 15 grams of fiber per day. This will gradually increase your total fiber intake in a GP-friendly way and boost the nutritional quality of your diet.

 Please note that fiber supplements are typically not recommended for GPers.

Live Well Tip: Managing Constipation

Constipation becomes an issue for many people with gastroparesis, most often due to a combination of diet and lifestyle factors. Managing constipation is essential for gastroparesis management, as constipation itself can exacerbate symptoms such as bloating, pain, and nausea. Chronic constipation may also further delay gastric emptying.

If you're struggling with constipation, here are some tips:

- **Drink more water:** even mild dehydration can lead to constipation since dry stools are more difficult to pass. It's important to drink an adequate amount of water and other non-caffeinated beverages each day (caffeine causes the body to eliminate fluid, thereby contributing to dehydration). If drinking a full glass of water makes you feel full or otherwise symptomatic, try keeping a water bottle with you and taking small sips consistently throughout the day.

- **Be more active:** physical activity helps to alleviate constipation by decreasing the amount of time it takes for stool to move through the colon. Regular exercise is also important for overall gastroparesis management, so aim for a total of at least 30 minutes of mild to moderate activity each day (see page 97).

- **Reduce processed food:** a low-fat, low-fiber diet consisting primarily of processed and packaged food is likely to lead to constipation. Try slowly replacing *some* of the refined food in your diet with GP-friendly fruits and vegetables, keeping your personal fiber tolerance in mind. Note that you *must* drink more water as you increase your intake of fruits and veggies or you may become even more constipated.

- **Don't ignore the urge:** when you have to go, go! Ignoring the urge to have a bowel movement may eventually result in the absence of urges, leading to chronic constipation.

- **Talk with your doctor:** certain medications, including some antiemetics and most narcotic pain relievers, can cause or worsen constipation. Discuss alternative options with your doctor. Your doctor may also recommend over-the-counter laxatives such as Miralax to treat constipation.

While constipation among people with gastroparesis is *most often* the result of diet and lifestyle factors, in some cases there are underlying conditions such as hypothyroidism, which contribute to both gastroparesis and chronic constipation. Other possibilities include dysmotility in the colon and/or pelvic floor dysfunction, a condition in which the muscles around the rectum don't relax properly to allow stool to pass. Always discuss any changes in your bowel habits with your doctor to ensure proper diagnosis and treatment.

Should I avoid anything labeled "whole-grain?"

The phrase "Made with Whole Grains!" is plastered on all kinds of packaged foods these days, though it usually has more to do with marketing than with nutrition. Most of these products are made with *whole grain flour,* which is not the same as *a whole grain.* Flour is completely pulverized and in many cases the fibrous part of the grain has been removed. Therefore, some whole grain flours are actually gastroparesis-friendly.

If you see a product that claims that it's made with whole grains, it doesn't mean you can't eat it. It just means you have to do a little detective work. First, check the fiber content listed on the nutrition panel. Then check the ingredient list. Look for anything that's *not* GP-friendly: nuts, seeds, rolled oats, or dried fruits, for example. If both of these things check out, regardless of the "whole grain" claim, it's likely to be GP-friendly.

How much fiber mentioned on the nutritional panel is too much?

Just like the total amount of fiber per day, the amount of fiber tolerated at any one time varies from person to person. In general, if a product has three or fewer grams of fiber per serving, it may be well tolerated. The caveat here, of course, is that you have to stay mindful of serving sizes and think about how many servings you're likely to eat at one time. Eat a cup and a half of a cereal with three grams of fiber per ¾ cup serving and you've eaten six grams of fiber: almost half of your daily maximum!

I've noticed that a lot of products have added fiber. Is that a problem?

Fiber is creeping up everywhere these days, from jelly to yogurt to ice cream. Manufacturers are adding chemical fiber, in the form of inulin, malodextrin, and polydextrose, to formerly (and naturally) fiber-free foods in an effort to make them appear healthier. If a product says it is low-fat and low-sugar, it's a safe bet that there's added fiber. This "stealth fiber" presents a few problems for GPers.

First, you need to have a general idea of how much fiber you're eating in order to adequately manage gastroparesis. Consuming products with added fiber can cause your symptoms to flare up without your even knowing why. (Remember, the average GPer tolerates about 10–15 grams of fiber per day.) *10-15 grams Fiber* *avoid*

In addition, the fiber that's added to these products is produced in a lab...not by nature. These additives are even harder on the GI tract than natural fiber and can exacerbate bloating, gas, cramping, and pain.

Lastly, because fiber is limited in a gastroparesis diet, you want to ensure that you're getting your allotment from nutritious foods such as fruits, veggies, and minimally processed grains—not from "fiber-fortified" junk foods that do nothing to promote good health.

How do I know if something has fiber added to it?

GPers have to be detectives of a sort when deciding which foods to buy. Before you put something in your cart—even if it's usually GP-friendly or you've eaten it in the past—check out the nutrition label *and* ingredient list. If it contains artificial fiber, you'll usually see inulin, malodextrin, or polydextrose listed.

I don't feel that great in the morning. Can I just skip breakfast?

Eating breakfast is important for a number of reasons. Our bodies need a certain number of calories (energy) to function. If you don't feed your body early in the day, it will demand extra fuel later on. If you skip breakfast, you may notice increased desire later in the day to keep eating after you're full or to snack frequently, or you may experience cravings for energy-dense foods that are high in fat or sugar, especially in the afternoon or evening. Forgoing a morning meal can also contribute to weight issues (either in gain or loss, depending on your metabolism, dieting history, and other circumstances) and it can compromise your overall nutrition.

Skipping breakfast generally sets up and perpetuates a cycle that looks like this: you skip breakfast, eat the majority of your food in the afternoon and evening, wake up the next morning feeling full and sick (because all the food you ate the previous afternoon and evening sat in your stomach while you slept), so you skip breakfast and start all over again. The good news is that when you break the cycle of eating the majority of your food in the evening and instead spread it throughout the entire day (starting with a well-balanced breakfast), you're likely to see an improvement in your morning symptoms and overall nutrition.

Live Well Tip: Eat a Well-Balanced Breakfast

I encourage all GPers to eat a well-balanced breakfast containing protein, carbohydrates, and a small amount of healthy fat whenever possible. A breakfast high in carbs and low in protein can lead to reactive hypoglycemia, or low blood sugar, even in non-diabetics. This is especially true for people with gastroparesis due to the erratic emptying of the stomach. Hypoglycemia can cause symptoms such as shakiness, dizziness, sweating, headache, and mental fogginess, and may trigger cravings for sugar and other carbohydrates. Erratic blood sugar may also affect the rate of gastric emptying over time.

Here are some examples of well-balanced gastroparesis-friendly breakfasts:

- Fruit smoothie made with unsweetened almond milk and 1 scoop of protein powder

- Cream of brown rice made with unsweetened soy milk, mixed with 4 ounces pureed fruit and 1 tablespoon of smooth almond butter

- 1 egg, 1 slice of Canadian bacon, and 1 ounce low-fat cheese on a toasted white English muffin

- 1 carton of Orgain Meal Replacement beverage (see page 63)

- 6 ounces 2% vanilla Greek yogurt; 1/2 sliced banana; 1/2 cup Rice Chex

- 6 ounces 0% Greek yogurt mixed with 1 tablespoon creamy peanut butter and a dash of cinnamon; 1 banana

- 1 slice of toast spread with 1 tablespoon of smooth cashew butter; 8 ounces protein-rich beverage

What does a "low-fat" diet mean?

As with fiber, the more dietary fat in a meal, the longer that meal will take to empty from the stomach. This true for everyone, regardless of whether or not they have gastroparesis. Following a low-fat diet helps food to empty as quickly as possible, thereby alleviating symptoms.

Low-fat, however, does not mean no fat. We need some dietary fat in order for our bodies to function properly. On average, a gastroparesis-friendly diet includes between 25 and 45 grams of fat per day. While some people tolerate slightly less and some people tolerate a little more, this tends to be the range at which most people notice a reduction in their symptoms yet can still obtain adequate nutrition and calories from fat. Fat has more than twice as many calories per gram than either carbohydrates or protein, so overly restricting the fat in your diet can lead to unintended weight loss.

What if I tolerate something that's higher in fat? Can I still eat it?

While eating too much fat can exacerbate your symptoms, it won't make your gastroparesis worse overall. In fact, many GPers tolerate higher fat foods (such as nut butter or avocado) in moderation as part of a well-managed GP-friendly diet. There's no need to exclude these foods completely unless they make you feel worse. Likewise, if you notice that you tolerate more than 45-50 grams of fat per day without feeling too full or symptomatic to meet your nutrition needs, there's no need to further restrict your intake.

How much fat should I eat at one time?

It's generally best to divide up your fat intake throughout the day. So, for example, if you eat six times per day and you tolerate between 40 and 45 grams of fat, you'd want to aim for about 7 grams of fat at each meal. You may find that you tolerate slightly more fat in the morning or in the evening, depending on when you're least symptomatic. Adjust your intake accordingly.

7 grams fat per meal

Be careful, though. While a higher-fat meal may not make you symptomatic immediately, it may enhance fullness and provoke symptoms at subsequent meals. Again, you have to be a bit of a detective in these situations. If, for example, you're too full at dinnertime, look at your meals earlier in the day to see how much fat (and fiber) you're taking in at each. You may need to tweak your lunch or afternoon snack(s). On the flip side, if you're too full at breakfast time, consider what you're eating for dinner and try changing up the composition of your evening meals.

What kinds of fat are GP-friendly?

Pretty much any kind of fat is GP-friendly. It's the *amount* of fat that you need to be most concerned about. Olive oil, canola oil, and butter, for example, can all be included in a gastroparesis diet so long as they are used in small amounts. A tablespoon of butter contains 11 grams of fat and a tablespoon of oil has about 14 grams of fat, so a GP-friendly serving is about one to two teaspoons of either.

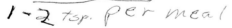
1-2 tsp. per meal

Are there any high-fat foods I should avoid altogether?

You should avoid fried foods and fatty meats, because these are almost guaranteed to provoke symptoms. In addition, they are not health promoting and do little to nourish your body. Trans fat should also be eliminated from your diet. Trans fats are manufactured substances found in many packaged and processed foods. Research shows that trans fats can increase "bad" (LDL) cholesterol, lower "good" (HDL) cholesterol, and increase your risk of cardiovascular disease. Note that products can contain as much as .49 grams of trans fat *per serving* and still be labeled "No Trans Fats." Check the ingredient list. If you see hydrogenated or partially hydrogenated oils, skip it.

Are full-fat liquids GP-friendly?

For some people, fat is better tolerated in liquid form. Full-fat dairy products like milkshakes and ice cream, for example, may not exacerbate symptoms. This isn't universally true for all GPers, though, so you'll have to experiment to see whether or not it works for you. Remember, eating foods that are higher in fat will not make gastroparesis more severe overall, so it's okay to do this kind of experimentation. If you do tolerate full-fat liquids, they can be especially helpful for maintaining or gaining weight. Just keep in mind that that if you experience increased fullness or other symptoms, you may need to reduce fat even in liquid form.

Is it best to follow an all-liquid diet?

In general, liquids empty from the stomach more quickly than solids. In fact, even in patients with no motility, liquids will often leave the stomach by gravity alone. That said, the typical gastroparesis-friendly diet includes a variety of solid foods in addition to purees, soft foods, and liquids. It is a small minority of patients who cannot tolerate any solid food and must consistently rely on an all-liquid diet.

What role do liquids play in a healthy gastroparesis diet?

While completely eliminating solid foods from the diet typically isn't necessary in order to manage gastroparesis, liquids can have an important role in the diet. During flare-ups, for example, switching to an all-liquid diet may help alleviate symptoms and give the GI tract a chance to fully empty and rest.

Liquids can also help increase caloric intake and prevent weight loss, especially when alternated with solid meals. To support proper nutrition, avoid "empty" liquids—things like regular and diet soda, fruit punch, and sports drinks. Opt for healthier choices like coconut water, 100% fruit and vegetable juices, pureed soups, smoothies, and organic meal replacement drinks.

How do I know when to eat solid meals and when to choose liquids?

Finding the best meal pattern takes a bit of experimentation, but it can make a big difference in terms of symptom management. In general, there are two approaches.

The first is to simply alternate every other meal between solid and liquid/soft foods. This coincides well with "normal" mealtimes, as you can eat breakfast, lunch, and dinner, and have smoothies, soups, purees or meal replacement drinks for your snacks in between. This will allow extra time for the solid food to empty between mealtimes without compromising calories or nutrition.

The second type of meal plan is based upon your least symptomatic time of the day. For example, if you feel better in the morning, you may eat solid food for your first three meals and then switch over to liquids or soft foods for your final three or four meals of the day. If you feel better toward evening, then you'd do the reverse.

Live Well Tip: Design Your Own Meal Plan

Meal Pattern Experiment

Try this easy two-week experiment to figure out the meal pattern that works best for you. Keep track of your daily symptom score in a food journal as you go.

Week One: Eat 1 cup (8 ounces) of gastroparesis-friendly food every 2 hours.

Week Two: Eat 1.5 cups (12 ounces) of gastroparesis-friendly food every 4 hours.

Which worked better for you? _____

Meal Composition Experiment

This two-week experiment will help you determine the meal composition that works best for you. Follow the meal pattern that you found worked best for you in the previous experiment.

Week One: Alternate liquid and solid meals/snacks throughout the day. For example, have solid or semi-solid food for breakfast, lunch and dinner, and smoothies, pureed soups, or meal replacement drinks as snacks in between.

Week Two: If you tend to feel best in the morning, eat solid food for the first 3-4 meals of the day and switch to liquids for the last 3-4 meals. If you're less symptomatic in the evening, reverse the pattern.

Which worked better for you? _____

Your Meal Pattern & Composition

Based on what you discovered during these four weeks, place a check mark next to the meals/snacks that make you feel better. Circle whether you do better with liquids or solids at that particular meal. Remember, this is just a guide. It's not carved in stone and may change over time.

    o Breakfast: solid   liquid ✓

    o A.M. Snack 1:   solid   liquid

    o A.M. Snack 2:   solid   liquid

    o Lunch: solid   liquid

    o P.M. Snack 1:   solid   liquid

> o P.M. Snack 2:   solid   liquid
>
> o Dinner: solid   liquid
>
> o Evening Snack: solid   liquid

Should I adhere to an all-liquid diet during a flare up?

When you're especially symptomatic, following a full liquid diet can help to alleviate your symptoms while still providing you with the calories and nutrition that your body needs to function.

In addition to thin liquids like juice and broth, a full liquid diet typically includes:

- Thin fruit, vegetable, or meat purees

- Thin, hot cereal (Cream of Wheat, Cream of Rice, Farina, etc.)

- Thin, creamy mashed potatoes   *Turnips*

- Smoothies

- Pureed soups

- Meal replacement drinks

- Yogurt

- Gelatin

- Ice cream, sherbet, frozen yogurt

Should I be using meal replacement drinks as part of my diet?

Many GPers rely on meal replacement/nutritional supplement drinks as staples in their diet. Because they're calorically dense, these drinks can be quite useful if you're having a hard time maintaining your weight, especially when consumed as a snack between existing meals.

Meal replacement drinks also tend to be fortified with vitamins and minerals, so regular consumption can help improve overall nutrition. While most of the nutrients found in these beverages are chemically added and therefore not as readily absorbed as those found in whole foods, they are better than nothing.

These products also come in handy when you're traveling or eating on the go. If you always have one on hand, all you'll need is a glass of ice to make a well-balanced GP-friendly meal. (I always have an Orgain in my purse and one in my car…just in case!)

Keep in mind that these drinks do contain fat (anywhere from 4 grams up to 15 or more grams per serving depending on the brand) and some contain several grams of fiber. That needs to be factored into your daily totals.

How do I choose a meal replacement drink?

Out of all of the meal replacement drinks currently on the market, Orgain is my personal favorite. Based on the nutritional content and the quality of ingredients, it's also the one I feel most comfortable recommending to my clients. (I have no affiliation with the company.)

One consideration is the high amount of sugar in many of these products, which some GPers find leads to cravings for more sweets, negatively impacts their mood, or has other undesirable effects. Boost and Ensure both contain between 22 and 27 grams of sugar per 8-ounce serving, depending on the flavor. That's about 6 teaspoons of sugar. Ready-to-drink Carnation Instant Breakfast has a whopping 39 grams of sugar. That's nearly 10 teaspoons—more than a Hershey bar! Carnation Instant Breakfast powder has 19 grams of sugar before you add the milk, which bumps the sugar content to about 30 grams total. Orgain has by the least sugar by far with 13 grams (about 3 teaspoons) per 11 ounce serving.

When choosing a meal replacement drink, it's important to take a look at the ingredients. Many contain artificial sweeteners like sucralose (Splenda), aspartame, and acesulfame potassium. The reason these substances have no calories is because your body can't digest or absorb them. Unfortunately, they often cause symptoms like bloating, pain, cramping, diarrhea, and gas as they pass through the GI tract undigested.

Some drinks also contain added fiber in the form of inulin or fructo-oligosaccharides (FOS). These are chemically-produced fibers that are also known to cause bloating, gas, cramping, pain, and nausea in some people. If you're using meal replacement drinks to manage your symptoms, especially during flare-ups, and you don't notice any improvement, some of these ingredients may be to blame.

Orgain doesn't contain any artificial sweeteners or added fiber. It does contain an ingredient called carrageenan, which some studies have suggested is carcinogenic in large quantities. Unfortunately, carrageenan is found in nearly all meal replacement drinks to improve texture and mouth-feel. While carrageenan is not something we want to be consuming too much of, I'm still comfortable drinking and recommending Orgain—especially given the alternatives.

Obviously, none of this matters if you can't tolerate the product. A lot of people will find they tolerate either Boost or Ensure, but not both. Some can't tolerate either. Many of my clients who had a hard time with other products have found that Orgain settles very well for them. However, it does contain some lactose, so it might not be appropriate if you're lactose-intolerant. Boost, Ensure, and Enlive are lactose free, though they do contain milk protein and are not appropriate for those on a dairy-free diet.

I've tried meal replacement drinks, but I seem to have trouble tolerating them. What can I do?

While liquids in general empty more quickly than solids, nutrient-dense liquids empty more slowly than other liquids. If you find that meal replacement drinks exacerbate your symptoms, try diluting them with up to equal parts water.

If regurgitation is an issue, make an effort to drink more slowly, one sip at a time, and hold each sip in your mouth for a few seconds to allow digestion to begin. These simple steps may make a significant difference in your ability to hold down these drinks.

Here's how I use Orgain: in a BPA-free 20-ounce water bottle, I mix half a carton of Orgain and six to eight ounces of water, then fill to the top with ice. I carry this around with me and sip on the diluted drink all day. I typically refill the bottle in the afternoon and again in the evening, meaning I drink one and a half cartons of Orgain per day. Drinking it this way, diluted and sipped slowly over the course of the day, doesn't fill me up or exacerbate my symptoms.

Live Well Tip: How You Eat Matters, Too

What you eat is important, but so is *how* you eat. Stress of any kind activates the sympathetic nervous system. The sympathetic nervous system is responsible for what most of us know as the "fight or flight" response. When your body goes into "fight or flight" mode, it shuts down any unnecessary processes, including digestion. So eating while stressed or anxious can actually exacerbate your symptoms, regardless of what you're eating. On the other hand, when you eat in a relaxed manner (when you are not feeling stressed or anxious), that allows the parasympathetic nervous system to remain in control, which facilitates digestion. Avoid eating in your car or on the go whenever possible. Don't discuss stressful or contentious topics over meals. Make the environment as relaxing and enjoyable as possible.

When you're relaxed during mealtimes, you also tend to slow down. Eating too quickly makes you more likely to eat more than you can tolerate, so you may wind up feeling overly full. It also makes you less likely to be satisfied with smaller, gastroparesis-friendly portions. Since portions are small to begin with, when you gobble them down quickly, your brain doesn't have time to even realize that you're eating. You wind up feeling full physically, but unsatisfied mentally. To practice eating more slowly and increase satisfaction, take the time to look at and smell your food before you eat it. Put your utensils down between bites or your glass down between sips. And chew.

While most of us don't give much thought to chewing, it's actually quite important when it comes to managing gastroparesis.

When you start to chew, it signals the stomach to ready itself for food by increasing the digestive juices. Chewing also reduces the workload of the stomach by breaking food into smaller pieces, which are easier to grind and empty. In addition, there are enzymes in the mouth that break down carbohydrates as we chew. So if you neglect to chew our food adequately, you actually start the digestive process off at a disadvantage.

Making an effort to chew every single bite thoroughly, until it's nearly a liquid, can have a significant impact on symptoms. I even recommend "chewing" your liquids! When you take a sip, hold it in your mouth for a few seconds so that the enzymes in the saliva can begin their work.

What can I do about food-related anxiety?

If you're feeling anxious when it comes to eating, it's something that needs to be addressed. Though it's common and understandable, the anxiety itself can exacerbate and intensify symptoms like nausea, vomiting, fullness or pain.

In addition to exacerbating symptoms, food-related anxiety usually leads to an overly restricted diet. Rather than risk symptoms, you may find yourself relying on a handful of "safe" staples, eating the same foods day in and day out. Not only is this mentally unsatisfying, it also compromises nutrition and often results in a variety of secondary issues, like vitamin and mineral deficiencies.

Remember that dietary modifications are not the only tool you have for symptom management. In fact, a GP-friendly diet is only one part of your comprehensive management plan. Integrating the other aspects of symptom management, including physical activity, stress reduction, appropriate medical treatment, and/or complementary therapies, can have a significant impact on the amount and variety of foods you're able to tolerate.

This means that the first step to overcoming food-related anxiety is to begin putting your comprehensive management plan into action. As your symptoms are better managed overall, you'll find that your ability to venture outside of your "safe" food zone increases. Careful and consistent experimentation is essential, both to increase your comfort with eating in general and your confidence with trying new foods.

I often recommend that my clients try one new gastroparesis-friendly food each week and keep track of their progress in a food journal. This journal allows you to see how your symptoms relate to the foods that you eat over time. While you probably won't tolerate everything that you try, you may be able to eat more foods than you realize. Also keep in mind that if you eat something that does cause symptoms, it will not do any long-term harm. In other words, eating something that does not agree with you will not make the gastroparesis more severe overall. Sometimes this knowledge alone helps to put the mind at ease.

If none of these things prove helpful or the anxiety is severe, consult a mental health professional. Food-related anxiety is common among people with gastroparesis, but it must be addressed in order to achieve adequate symptom management and overall nutrition. Talking with a trained professional in a safe, non-judgmental environment can be extremely beneficial.

Is it necessary to keep a food journal if I eat the same things all the time?

Keeping a food journal is one of the best ways to figure out what works for you and what doesn't. When you're experimenting with new foods, it's important to have a written record, because our memories aren't nearly as good as we think. A journal also allows you to track your symptoms over time and to see whether they're getting better, worse, or are staying the same as you're making changes to your diet and other aspects of your symptom management plan.

Keeping a food journal can help prevent over-restriction, as well. Oftentimes we end up with a list of "safe" foods, but we've forgotten about other foods that we have eaten and tolerated well in the past. Your food journal provides a complete record of the foods that you've been able to tolerate, as well as the ones that haven't worked well for you. Sometimes a certain food might be causing symptoms, but because it's GP-friendly, you don't necessarily recognize it as an issue. A food journal makes these kinds of patterns much easier to identify.

What should I keep track of in my food journal?

The most important pieces of information for you to track are when and what you eat, including approximate portion sizes; any medications or supplements that you take; and any symptoms that you experience. You don't necessarily need to keep track of nutritional information like fat or fiber. In fact, sometimes paying *too* much attention to that kind of stuff can exacerbate anxiety and stress.

I also highly recommend that you record a daily symptom score. This means that at the end of each day, you rate your symptoms on a scale of 1–5. One represents a symptom-free day. Five indicates a severely symptomatic day.

The symptom score allows you to easily identify whether your symptoms are getting better, worse, or staying the same over time. This comes in very handy when you start making changes to your diet, supplementation plan, or other aspects of your management plan. It can also provide peace of mind during flare-ups. Sometimes symptoms seem to flare up for no apparent reason and you may worry that the gastroparesis itself has gotten worse. Taking a look at your symptom score over time will allow you to see that the ebb and flow of symptoms is a "normal" part of your journey with gastroparesis.

How many times should I try a new food before I rule it out, and how much should I try?

Trying a food only once isn't a very good indication of whether or not you tolerate it in general. That's because so many things contribute to the symptoms that you may experience: everything from what you've eaten earlier in the day, to the environment in which you eat, to the medications or supplements you've taken that day.

I typically advise my clients to try a food two or three times before deciding whether to keep or eliminate it as part of their diet. If you try something twice and it makes you ill both times, that's a fairly good indicator. If you eat it twice and the results are mixed, give it one more try.

As far as how much of a food to try, that depends on what you're eating. For higher-fat foods like nut butters, probably about a tablespoon would be sufficient. A new cereal, on the other hand? Maybe one half to one cup. Certainly the portion should be a gastroparesis-friendly one. For example, eating three cups of *anything* would likely cause symptoms.

Why do I feel hungry or have the urge to eat even when I know I'm full?

When the stomach empties slowly, it's very possible to feel both "hungry" and "full" at the same time. That's because though you've eaten and your stomach is full, the food hasn't yet been digested and absorbed. So your body is still asking for nutrients and energy, and your blood sugar may still be low. Depending on what you've already eaten, eating more could make you feel worse or exacerbate your symptoms later on. Sometimes simply drinking a small glass of 100% fruit juice will help alleviate the hunger, provide some energy, and raise your blood sugar.

Live Well Tip: Decoding FODMAPs

FODMAP is an acronym that stands for Fermentable Oligo-, Di-, and Mono-saccharides and Polyols. These FODMAPs are found in a variety of foods and cause a host of GI symptoms in susceptible people, especially those of us with FGIMDs. If it seems that regardless of what you eat, symptoms of bloating, belching and pain still plague you, it may be worth paying a little extra attention to FODMAPs in particular. Many of the foods that GPers come to think of as "safe" foods for gastroparesis-management are high in FODMAPs and could actually be *exacerbating* symptoms in some cases.

How can you identify the FODMAPs in your diet? Unfortunately, measuring the amount of FODMAPs in specific foods is still an emerging science and even the experts don't agree on all of the ins and outs of a low-FODMAP diet. But below is a list of foods known to be especially high in FODMAPs.

- Apples

- Pears

- Peaches

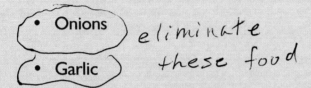

- Mangoes

- High-fructose corn syrup

- Honey

- Onions *eliminate these food*

- Garlic

- Artificial sweeteners ending in "ol" (read labels!)

- Dairy products (except for hard cheeses)

- Wheat products (bread, pasta, crackers, etc.)

Pay close attention to your symptoms when you eat these foods. Even better, try reducing or eliminating them and see if you feel any better.

Further Reading: *The Complete IBS Health & Diet Guide* by Dr. Maitreyi Raman, MD, MSc, FRCPC.

So with all of this in mind, how do I know exactly what to eat?

The bottom line is that there is no one-size-fits-all diet for gastroparesis. The only way to figure out *exactly* what works for you and what doesn't is careful and consistent experimentation based on the guidelines and information presented in this section. With the help of your food journal, you will begin to identify the foods and meal patterns that best alleviate your symptoms.

NUTRITION & SUPPLEMENTATION

If we're not willing to settle for junk living, we certainly shouldn't settle for junk food.

−Sally Edwards

It's impossible to overstate the importance of nutrition in a gastroparesis management plan. While a healthy body needs adequate nutrition in order to function properly, it's even *more* essential for those of us with chronic illness. Lack of nutrition makes it very difficult for the body to heal, repair, or even maintain the status quo in these situations. In fact, I believe that much of what is regarded as a progression of gastroparesis or a general degradation of health after a gastroparesis diagnosis may often be related to poor nutrition over time.

The goal is not necessarily perfect nutrition via diet alone. Obviously, that would be ideal, but given the dietary modifications that are necessary for symptom management, it's not possible in most cases. What we *can* do is make the most nutritious choices possible from our GP-friendly options and use nutritional supplements to fill in the gaps.

Do I have to be concerned about nutrition if I'm not losing weight?

Nutrition is about much more than weight. Malnutrition can be present whether you're underweight, overweight, or somewhere in between. It's certainly possible to consume enough calories to maintain your weight without obtaining adequate nutrients. While many medical professionals pay more attention to nutritional status in patients who are underweight or at risk of becoming underweight, I think it should be a consideration for every single person with gastroparesis.

How can I pay attention to nutrition if I have to limit my diet in order to manage symptoms?

Remember that dietary modifications are not the only tool for symptom management. In fact, the entire first half of this book is about managing your symptoms. Every section represents a different aspect of a comprehensive gastroparesis management plan. Dietary modifications are just one piece of that plan. On the flip side, there's really only one way to provide our bodies with adequate nourishment, and that's by making smart choices about what we put in our mouths.

You need to choose the foods that provide as much nourishment as possible without exacerbating symptoms. In other words, choose nutrient-dense, gastroparesis-friendly foods over nutritionally empty foods that simply take up space. As you read this section and begin to experiment, you'll likely find that there are nutrient-rich options that you tolerate just as well as the empty foods.

It's important to make only one change at a time so that you can identify what works for you and what doesn't. Making too many changes too quickly will almost certainly cause your symptoms to flare up. Small changes will add up over time to improve your nutrition without compromising symptom management.

How do I know if I'm getting proper nutrition?

Our bodies need a variety of vitamins and minerals, as well a balance of carbohydrates, protein, and fat in order to function properly. If your diet doesn't include a variety of foods, including fruits, vegetables, healthy fats, and lean protein, then you're likely not obtaining adequate nutrition. Put another way, if you're following a gastroparesis-friendly diet that's made up primarily of processed carbohydrates, you're most likely not getting the nutrients your body needs.

If you're concerned about your nutritional status, you may ask your doctor to run some common blood tests every 6–12 months, such as:

- Lipids

- CBC (Complete Blood Count)

- CMP (Comprehensive Metabolic Panel)

- Total protein

- Albumin

✓ Prealbumin (which is decreased in cases of malnutrition; it rises and falls rapidly in response to treatment)

• Iron tests (such as Iron, TIBC, and Ferritin)

• Specific vitamins and minerals (such as B_{12} and Folate, Vitamin D, Vitamin K, Calcium, and Magnesium)

Live Well Tip: Baby Food is Just Puree

You may have heard of people with gastroparesis eating baby food. While that probably sounds unappealing or even depressing, what most of us call "baby food" is really just pureed fruits and vegetables. For GPers, such purees can allow you to incorporate more fruits and vegetables into your diet, including things that you're unable to eat in whole form like peas, green beans, and berries.

You can either buy the purees (sold as "baby food") or make your own (see page 179 for tips). I don't recommend making purees that include peas, beans, corn, or berries unless you have a Vitamix or similar high-end appliance. Buying baby food versions of these foods will ensure that the indigestible parts have been removed. Buy organic commercial baby food whenever possible to avoid pesticides and chemicals, since any that are used during growing processes become concentrated in purees.

Whole Foods

Here's a tip: don't eat commercial baby food straight out of the jar. Nobody is happy sitting at the dinner table eating out of a jar. At least put it in a fancy dish. Also keep in mind that you don't have to eat puree on its own. Purees can be used in a variety of ways to increase the nutrient quality of what you're already eating. Try mixing vegetable puree into mashed

> potatoes, soups, or pasta sauces. Stir pureed fruits into yo-gurt, cottage cheese, or hot cereals. Add them to smooth-ies or even other purees. Get creative! Of course, whether you're making or buying your purees, they do contain some fiber—so you want to go slowly when incorporating them into your diet and do so within your personal limits.

Is it okay to just stick to a few safe foods?

While it's common for people with gastroparesis to find and stick to a small number of "safe" foods, this isn't mentally satisfying or physically nourishing. Different foods offer different nutrients. If you're eating only a handful of foods, you're missing out on a lot of the nutrients that your body needs to function properly.

We were meant to eat a wide variety of foods in order to obtain the appropriate nutrients that our bodies need. In fact, nature builds variety into our diet in the form of seasonal foods. Traditionally, the food that was available to us changed depending on the time of the year. While large supermarkets now make seasonal eating less of a focus, it's still possible (and advisable!) to eat this way with gastroparesis by choosing GP-friendly fruits and vegetables that are in season.

How can I incorporate more variety in my diet?

Eating seasonally will increase diet variety throughout the year, but we should also strive for variety in our weekly and daily food intake. This will enhance overall nutrition, reduce the risk of specific vitamin and mineral deficiencies, mitigate the effects of less healthy choices, and prevent boredom and mental dissatisfaction.

One of the easiest ways to ensure that you're getting a variety of foods and nutrients in your diet is to eat foods in a variety of colors. Eat a rainbow of foods, in other words. Most of the typical gastroparesis-friendly diet looks pretty dull: lots of white, beige, and brown. But there are a number of brightly colored foods that are either naturally GP-friendly or can be prepared in GP-friendly ways, such as pureeing and juicing.

Live Well Tip: The GP-Friendly Rainbow

Red

- Beets: canned, juiced, or roasted

- Cherry juice

- Cranberry juice

- Pomegranate juice

- Roasted red peppers: pureed

- Tomato juice*

- Tomato sauce (strained)*

- Watermelon (seedless): raw or in smoothies

Yellow/Orange

- "Baby food" apricots or corn

- Cantaloupe: raw or in smoothies

- Carrots: juiced, steamed, roasted, or pureed

- Lemons*: juiced

- Mango: in smoothies or pureed

- Peaches: canned, cooked, in smoothies, or pureed

- Pumpkin: canned or pureed

- Sweet Potatoes: baked, roasted, or pureed

- Turmeric (natural anti-inflammatory and painkiller): spice

- Winter Squash: pureed or in soup

Green:

- Avocado (in small amounts): raw, in smoothies or soups

- "Baby food" peas and green beans

- Celery: juiced *ck iron*

- Cucumber: juiced

- Green juices: Bolthouse Farms, Naked Juice

- Green tea

- Honeydew: raw or in smoothies

- Spinach: well-cooked and/or pureed, or in smoothies

Blue/Purple

- Acai juice

- "Baby food" blueberries, plums, and prunes

- Blueberry juice *?*

- Grape juice

- Purple carrots: steamed, roasted, or pureed

- Purple potatoes: mashed, boiled, baked, or roasted

White

- Bananas: raw, in smoothies, or pureed

- Cauliflower: mashed, pureed, or in soup *ck iron*

- Coconut milk (light)

- Coconut water

- Ginger (natural antiemetic): tea, spice, etc.

- Mushrooms: cooked

- Parsnips: mashed, pureed, or roasted

- Pears: canned, stewed, or pureed

- Potatoes: mashed, boiled, baked, or roasted

- White grape juice

If you have GERD or acid reflux, these foods may exacerbate your symptoms.

Is it okay to stick to mostly carbohydrates to manage symptoms?

While the typical gastroparesis diet lacks color, most also lack a healthy balance of carbohydrates, protein, and fat. Each of these three macronutrients is important to overall health and has specific functions within the body.

Carbohydrates are the body's main source of fuel (energy). They can be used immediately or stored for later use. The brain, central nervous system, kidneys, and the muscles all need carbohydrates in order to function. The gastroparesis diet tends to be very heavy in carbohydrates but lacking in protein and healthy fats.

Protein is found in every living cell in the body. It's essential for building and maintaining bones, muscles and skin, as well as making hormones. Protein is also necessary for tissue repair and proper immune function.

Fat is important for normal growth and development, as well as maintaining cell membranes and cushioning the internal organs. Fat is required for proper absorption of vitamins A, D, E, and K, as well as carotenoids. Women also need adequate amounts of fat to regulate their menstrual cycle.

The ideal amount of protein, carbohydrates and fat varies from person to person based on a number of factors—everything from age and sex to ancestry and blood type. This is called bio-individuality. For those on a gastroparesis diet, the optimal breakdown tends to be about 55 to 70 percent carbohydrates, 10 to 25 percent protein, and 10 to 20 percent fat.

How do I find out what works best for me and how closely should I follow this ratio?

Figuring out the right proportions for you may take some experimentation. On the other hand, you may know from your time prior to gastroparesis whether you tended to thrive on more protein or more carbohydrates, and so on.

You don't really need to count or keep track of your percentages. The key is to make sure that all your meals and snacks contain a variety of carbs, protein, and little bit of fat. If you're having a hard time managing your blood sugar, you may be eating too many carbohydrates. Adding a little protein and/or fat will often help correct the issue (see page 84).

How can I boost the protein in my diet?

Protein can pose issues for those with impaired digestion, since it requires more energy, enzymes, and acids to break down than do carbohydrates. However, as you've read, it's a vital part of a healthy, well-balanced diet.

Eggs are an easy-to-digest, versatile source of protein. While many GPers stick to egg whites in order to reduce fat, most of the nutrients are in the yolk. A large egg, yolk and all, has less than 5 grams of fat — about the same as a half tablespoon of peanut butter. In terms of cholesterol, having one to two eggs per day isn't an issue for most people.

Try adding an egg to one of your mini-meals, whether it's scrambled with your usual piece of toast for breakfast or hard boiled alongside the crackers you typically eat for a snack, to increase the protein by seven grams and bump up the total nutrition in the meal.

Lean animal protein, though more difficult to digest, is certainly GP-friendly for those who can tolerate it. Skinless chicken breast, turkey breast, lean ground turkey, lean ground beef, ground bison, and wild game such as venison are all lower-fat, high-protein choices. Some GPers may also tolerate poultry sausage and hot dogs.

protein?

The majority of the protein in many gastroparesis diets comes from low-fat dairy products such as milk, yogurt, cheese, and cottage cheese. Greek yogurt in particular is a fantastic source of dairy protein—it's nearly equivalent to a three-ounce serving of chicken breast! Keep in in mind that dairy products may exacerbate certain GI symptoms, even if you're not lactose-intolerant. If you notice increased bloating, belching, gas or pain after eating milk, ice cream or other dairy products, try reducing your consumption in favor of other protein-rich GP-friendly choices. Note that hard cheeses such as Parmesan may still be well tolerated.

Creamy nut butters are a satisfying, nutrient-rich source of vegetarian protein. While they're high in fat, a little bit goes a long way. About two tablespoons of creamy nut butter per day is usually well tolerated as part of a GP-friendly diet. Without taking up much space, it can bump up the protein content and overall nutrition value of an otherwise empty snack like graham crackers, pretzels, or toast. If you find that peanut butter exacerbates your symptoms, try almond butter or cashew butter instead. Whereas peanuts are a legume, cashews and almonds are tree nuts and are often well tolerated.

✱ hard to digest

Soy, while also a good source of vegetarian protein, can be difficult to digest. Traditionally, soy has been consumed in fermented products such as miso and tempeh. Most of the soy products on the market today, including soy milk, yogurt, and ice cream, are highly processed and may exacerbate stomach pain and other symptoms. If you do well with soy products, they can be a useful alternative to dairy.

Live Well Tip: Finding the Right Protein Supplements

Protein powders and protein bars can come in handy as part of a well-balanced gastroparesis diet, especially for those who cannot tolerate animal protein or who choose to follow a vegetarian diet. These are processed foods, however, so it's important to look for high-quality products with as few ingredients as possible.

Protein Powders

There are so many protein powders on the market that it's hard to know where to start. In general, most GPers will tolerate one of four types of protein:

- Whey—readily available and inexpensive. Avoid if you are sensitive to dairy; use caution if you are lactose-intolerant, since many whey products contain traces of lactose.

- Soy—a vegetarian protein. Can be difficult to digest; may cause gas, pain or bloating.

- Egg White—easy to digest; may be frothy. Avoid if you are allergic to eggs.

- Brown Rice—typically well tolerated; an incomplete protein, though often fortified with additional amino acids. Gritty texture; less protein per serving than other options.

When choosing a protein powder, check the fiber content and choose a product with no more than 3 grams per serving, unless you plan to use less than one serving at a time. Avoid products that contain artificial sweeteners, especially sugar alcohols, which may exacerbate symptoms.

Protein Bars

A lot of protein bars are packed with ingredients that are hard to digest. In general I've found that the mushier or chewier a bar is to start with, the better it seems to settle. I'm partial to MacroBars because they are minimally processed and contain only a handful of ingredients. MacroBars do contain pieces of nuts, which will not be appropriate for everyone; I choose to pick them out.

Other protein bars that are GP-friendly include:

- Genisoy Bars

- Luna Protein Bars (not regular Luna bars)

- Balance Bar Original (not Bare or Gold)

Of these, Luna Protein would be my first choice because it doesn't contain any artificial sweeteners or corn syrup, and the ingredients are not genetically modified and are at least partially organic. As with protein powders, avoid bars with sugar alcohols (check the nutrition facts), and bars with more than 3 grams of fiber. As always, make sure you *chew* your protein bars really well—even the mushy and chewy ones—to support digestion.

Do I need to worry about my blood sugar if I'm not diabetic?

Reactive hypoglycemia is quite common among non-diabetic GPers, probably due to the combination of an unbalanced diet and the erratic emptying of the stomach. When we eat refined or processed low-fiber carbohydrates in the absence of protein and fat, blood sugar rises very quickly. The body releases insulin in order to decrease the amount of sugar in the blood. In cases of reactive hypoglycemia, the amount of insulin released causes the blood sugar to dip too low.

How do I know I'm experiencing low blood sugar?

Symptoms of low blood sugar include fatigue, dizziness, light-headedness, sweating, heart palpitations, headache, nervousness, and irritability. Dips in blood sugar can also lead to increased appetite and cravings for sweets, thus perpetuating the cycle of highs and lows.

It's important to note that symptoms similar to hypoglycemia can be experienced in the absence of documented low blood sugar. Generally, a medical evaluation is done to determine whether symptoms are caused by hypoglycemia and whether symptoms resolve once blood sugar returns to normal. Further evaluation and treatment depends on the severity of symptoms.

How can I keep my blood sugar stable?   *meals 3 hrs apart*

The guidelines I've outlined for a gastroparesis-friendly diet correspond with the recommendations for reactive hypoglycemia. You should eat several small meals and snacks throughout the day, approximately three hours apart. Meals and snacks should be well balanced and include GP-friendly carbohydrates, protein, and a bit of healthy fat. Sugary foods should be limited, especially first thing in the morning or on an otherwise empty stomach. The key here is to avoid all-carbohydrate or high-sugar meals that cause your pancreas to pump out large amounts of insulin once the food is finally emptied from the stomach. Aside from alleviating the unpleasant symptoms of hypoglycemia, this may help to reduce your risk of insulin resistance and possibly type 2 diabetes in the future.

Live Well Tip: Get Your Fatty Acids

Our bodies need twenty different fatty acids, all of which come from two essential fatty acids: linolenic acids (omega-3s) and linoleic acid (omega-6s). These are called essential fatty acids because our body can't make them; we have to get them from the food we eat. In addition to being the building blocks of other fatty acids, omega-3 and omega-6 fatty acids play a role in the digestive process and are important for the regulation of metabolism.

The typical gastroparesis diet, much like the typical American diet in general, contains more than enough omega-6 fatty acids. What most of us are lacking is an adequate amount of omega-3 fatty acids. Signs of a fatty acid deficiency include excessive thirst, frequent urination, and dry hair and skin.

GP-friendly sources of omega-3 fatty acids include salmon, scallops, trout, cod, crab, lobster and tilapia, but most GPers require supplementation in order to obtain an adequate amount. There are a variety of omega-3 supplements available. Look for one that contains both DHA and EPA, either from fish or from vegetarian sources like algae. Vegetarian formulas are often easier to digest than fish oils. Flax seed oil is also a good source omega-3 fatty acids and may be well tolerated in small amounts.

Will switching to more processed foods lead to better management of GP symptoms?

Many people think that a gastroparesis-friendly diet has to be filled with packaged and processed foods. The truth is, there are a number of whole, unprocessed, or minimally-processed choices that are naturally GP-friendly or can be prepared in way that makes them

GP-friendly. While preparing these kinds of foods may take a little more work, it's worth the effort when it comes to nutrition and satisfaction.

Whole foods naturally contain vitamins, minerals, enzymes, and phytonutrients that our bodies need to function, and especially to strengthen and repair. Most processed foods have been stripped of nutrients. While certain vitamins and minerals may have been added back in, they're typically low-quality manufactured versions that the body doesn't absorb or utilize as well. Processed foods also tend to be higher in sugar and salt, and they often contain trans fats, artificial colors, preservatives, and added sweeteners.

While the goal is to ensure that your diet is as nourishing as possible, it's important to stay mindful of symptom management. It's likely that a well-balanced gastroparesis diet will still include some processed foods, so you need to make smart choices. Look for products that are minimally-processed and contain as few ingredients as possible. For example, if you find two different GP-friendly products where one has five ingredients and another has fifteen, go with the first.

Should I choose organic food?

While those of us with gastroparesis have to pay attention to the *kinds* of food we eat, the *quality* of the food we choose is also important. Choosing organic is one way to increase the quality of the food in your diet. The artificial chemicals, colors, and sweeteners, as well as pesticides, antibiotics, and hormones that are often found in conventional products and produce do not support health or healing. In fact, many of these ingredients promote inflammation and can further tax the digestive system.

While choosing organic foods will minimize your exposure to these things, it's not possible or economical in all situations. The foods that I recommend spending the extra effort and money to purchase organic are:

- Meat and poultry. Unlike commercially-raised animals, organically-raised animals are not treated with antibiotics or growth hormones and are fed organically-grown grain that's free of pesticides, chemical fertilizers, and meat by-products. Remember that what your meat eats, you eat (the same goes for milk and eggs).

- Eggs. Organic eggs come from chickens that are not treated with antibiotics and are given organically-grown, vegetarian feed.

- Dairy products. Organic dairy comes from cows that have not been treated with antibiotics or growth hormones and which are fed organically-grown feed.

- Certain produce. Some fruits and vegetables are "dirtier" than others when it comes to pesticide and fertilizer residue. These are called the "Dirty Dozen." (See below.)

- Baby food. Because baby food is made of condensed vegetables and fruit, the level of any chemicals found on the food (pesticides, antibiotics, hormones, etc.) is intensified.

Organic

- Anything you eat very frequently. Pesticides, chemicals, artificial sweeteners, artificial colors, and preservatives can add up with frequent exposure.*

Remember that organic junk food is still junk food. Cookies and frozen yogurt, for example, even if they're organic, are still treats and should be eaten only occasionally as part of an overall balanced diet.

Live Well Tip: Avoid the Dirty Dozen

"The Dirty Dozen" are produce items that have been found to contain the most pesticide and chemical residue. Simply washing or peeling these fruits and vegetables is not an adequate way to reduce exposure, as the toxins penetrate the skin and are absorbed by the flesh of the produce. Buy certified organic versions of these products whenever possible:

- Apples (for juice, sauce, or cooking)

- Bell peppers (for juicing)

- Celery (for juicing)

- Cherries (as juice)

- Grapes (as juice)

- Lettuce (typically not GP-friendly)

- Nectarines (as juice)

- Peaches (fresh, frozen, canned, or nectar)

- Pears (fresh, frozen, canned, or nectar)

- Potatoes (all varieties)

- Spinach (for juicing or cooking)

- Strawberries (for juicing)

Least Contaminated Produce

These items contain the lowest amount of chemical residue and/or are protected by a thick outer skin that is removed prior to eating. You may wish to buy conventional versions of these GP-friendly products to save money.

- Avocado

- Bananas

- Cantaloupe

- Mango

- Melon

- Onions

- Papaya

- Pineapples

- Sweet potatoes

I don't have much of an appetite. How can I avoid losing weight?

When fullness or lack of appetite is leading to weight loss, it's even more important to ensure that every bite and sip you take is as nutrient- and calorically dense as possible. This means avoiding "empty" foods, as well as those that contain a lot of air. Anything that's puffed, whipped, or fluffed, including puffed cereals, rice cakes, whipped yogurt, and double-churned ice cream, is likely to fill up your stomach without providing nearly enough nutrition. The same goes for snack foods like cookies and crackers as well as soda and diet drinks.

Better choices include smoothies, soups, mashed or pureed fruits and vegetables, Greek yogurt, and meal replacement drinks. Sipping high calorie liquids throughout the day, in addition to your regular meals, can also help increase overall calories and nutrition without exacerbating symptoms. Odwalla, Bolthouse Farms, and Naked juice drinks, for example, are often well tolerated.

Is it normal to gain weight with gastroparesis?

Most people assume that gastroparesis leads to weight loss. While that's true for many GPers, there are others who maintain or even gain weight, regardless of the severity of their symptoms. The effect that gastroparesis has on your weight is likely due in part to your body type, metabolism, and even your history of dieting. If you're a chronic or yo-yo dieter, for example, your body may be more prone to hanging onto weight despite the restricted gastroparesis diet.

While it seems counterintuitive, the gastroparesis diet can factor into weight gain, especially if you're grazing all day long on foods that are high in refined carbohydrates and low in fat and protein. Taking in *too few* calories and too little nutrition can also cause the body to go into what's commonly referred to as "starvation mode," slowing metabolism and preventing weight loss.

Thyroid function may also play a role in whether you lose, maintain, or gain weight with gastroparesis. Hypothyroidism can cause everything to slow down, including digestion and metabolism. People who have gastroparesis due to impaired thyroid function may actually gain weight despite eating very little. If you have idiopathic gastroparesis and are gaining weight, consider asking your doctor about hypothyroidism.

Gaining or even maintaining weight can present difficulties when it comes to obtaining adequate treatment for gastroparesis since some doctors tend to correlate a patient's weight with the severity of their condition. If your doctor is ignoring or dismissing your complaints based on your weight, I encourage you to be proactive in finding a doctor who can better evaluate the situation and offer adequate treatment.

Live Well Tip: Losing Weight with Gastroparesis

While many GPers struggle to maintain or gain weight, others find themselves in need of healthy weight loss. There are several things to address when it comes to losing weight with gastroparesis:

- Eat balanced meals: eating a low-fat, high-carbohydrate diet that's too low in protein can make it difficult to lose weight. A diet too high in refined carbohydrates can lead to swings in blood sugar, resulting in cravings and increased appetite regardless of GP symptoms.

- Focus on quality: Some ingredients found in conventional products, such as high-fructose corn syrup and artificial sweeteners, may contribute to weight gain. Choose whole foods such as GP-friendly fruits and veggies and lean proteins, as well as minimally-processed foods like hot cereals, nut butters, soups, smoothies, and juices.

- Reduce stress: chronic stress has been found to impair weight loss, as well as exacerbate gastroparesis symptoms making it difficult to choose more nutritionally dense foods.

- Get more sleep: lack of sleep can slow the metabolism as well as lead to cravings and overeating.

- Practice yoga: a regular yoga practice calms the mind, helps to prevent mindless eating, strengthens the body, reduces overall stress, and promotes more restful sleep.

> • Incorporate more physical activity: mild to moderate physical activity is beneficial both for weight management and for managing gastroparesis symptoms. Aim for at least 30 minutes of activity each day.

Should I take vitamins?

Vitamins and minerals are essential to human health, and each one has specific functions within the body. Due to soil degradation, fruits and vegetables have lower mineral content today than they did several decades ago. In addition, most of the produce in our supermarkets has been trucked across the country (or even flown in from across the world); vitamins have been lost in the process.

That means that even if we were able to eat a completely healthy, whole food diet, it would be difficult to obtain all of the necessary nutrients from our diets alone. Factor in the lack of variety and fresh food in a typical gastroparesis diet, and the potential for vitamin and mineral deficiencies is fairly high. In addition, some GPers may have impaired absorption of certain nutrients. For all of these reasons, most people with gastroparesis will likely benefit from a daily multivitamin/mineral supplement.

When selecting a multivitamin/mineral supplement, look for one that has the United States Pharmacopeia (USP) seal. This ensures that the ingredients and amounts stated on the label are accurate, that the product is free of contaminants, and that it was found to dissolve properly for optimal absorption. Chewable tablets, liquid formulations, or gummy vitamins are often better tolerated than tablets and capsules. Look for a product that does not contain artificial dyes, sweeteners, or flavors and take it with meals to prevent or minimize stomach upset and aid in absorption.

How do I know if I am deficient in certain vitamins or minerals?

Many of the symptoms that are often attributed to either a worsening of gastroparesis or to new unrelated conditions may actually be the result of vitamin and mineral deficiencies.

Your doctor can order blood work to look for specific deficiencies. Depending on the results, as well as your health history, you may benefit from other supplements in addition to a multivitamin/mineral. Be sure to inform your doctor(s) about all supplements that you're taking, including vitamins and minerals.

Supplements that may be particularly important for GPers are:

Labs *3-6-21* *Low* *D3*

- **Vitamin D**, which is necessary for bone health, proper calcium absorption, and immune function. Vitamin D deficiency has been indicated in over twenty common diseases. Vitamin D is fat soluble, so adequate dietary fat is required for proper absorption. Look for a supplement containing Vitamin D3, since Vitamin D2 is not well absorbed and is minimally effective. A 25-Hydroxy Vitamin D blood test is recommended to determine your current level of Vitamin D.

- **Magnesium** is essential for proper functioning of the nervous, muscular, and cardio-vascular systems. It also helps to regulate the bowel. Deficiency symptoms include anxiety, insomnia, irritability, muscle weakness or cramping, Restless Leg Syndrome, and irregular heartbeat. There are several kinds of magnesium available. Magnesium oxide is not well absorbed. A better option is magnesium citrate, which is typically well tolerated, easy to find, and fairly inexpensive.

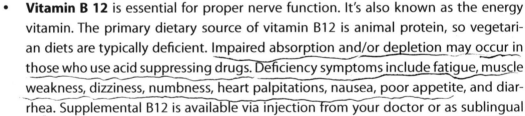
Sublingual B12

- **Vitamin B 12** is essential for proper nerve function. It's also known as the energy vitamin. The primary dietary source of vitamin B12 is animal protein, so vegetarian diets are typically deficient. Impaired absorption and/or depletion may occur in those who use acid suppressing drugs. Deficiency symptoms include fatigue, muscle weakness, dizziness, numbness, heart palpitations, nausea, poor appetite, and diarrhea. Supplemental B12 is available via injection from your doctor or as sublingual tablets. *Nexium ask Parrark*

An iron supplement is also necessary in some cases, but you should not take iron unless you have been told that you are iron deficient. Most men and post-menopausal women do not need supplemental iron. If you have symptoms of iron deficiency anemia, such as extreme fatigue, pale skin, weakness, shortness of breath, headache, dizziness or lightheadedness, cold hands and feet, inflammation or soreness of your tongue, brittle nails, or unusual cravings for ice or dirt, then you should ask your doctor to check the levels of iron and ferritin (iron stores) in your blood.

How do I know where to start with vitamin supplementation?

When introducing new supplements, it's important to try only one at a time. Wait several days, keeping track of any new or changing symptoms, before introducing the next product. This is the only way to determine exactly what does—and doesn't—work for you.

There are a wide variety of manufacturers and formulations for each vitamin/mineral listed. It may be necessary to experiment in order to find the one that's best for you. Chewable, sublingual, and liquid formulations are often better tolerated than tablets.

Unless otherwise directed by your doctor, start with the lowest dose possible and work your way up to determine the amount that's best tolerated. For example, if you're taking a multivitamin that has a dose of two tablets per day, you might start with one tablet a day for one week and then try two tablets per day the following week. If you have no trouble with one tablet, but find that two exacerbates your symptoms, some is better than none!

Live Well Tip: Blackstrap Molasses

If you are iron deficient but cannot tolerate iron supplements, either due to constipation or digestive upset, you might try blackstrap molasses. Blackstrap molasses is what's left over after cane sugar has been processed into table sugar. It's a good source of highly-absorbable:

- Iron

- Magnesium

- Copper

- Manganese

- Calcium

- Potassium

- Vitamin B6

Look for unsulfured blackstrap molasses, which is a purer product and is processed without chemicals. I recommend buying organic in this case, as well.

Try stirring a tablespoon of molasses directly into a mug of hot water or warm milk. The flavor is quite strong and may take some getting used to. If you find that it upsets your stomach, decrease the amount of molasses and/or dilute it in more liquid. You may find that you tolerate it better in the morning or afternoon than at the end of the day.

LIFESTYLE PRACTICES

Act as if what you do makes a difference. It does.

–William James

The lifestyle aspect of managing gastroparesis is often overlooked or underestimated. Some people think it's too simple a response for such a complicated problem. How could stress management or physical activity make a difference when all kinds of medication have failed? In actuality, the choices that you make in daily life matter a great deal. Lifestyle practices can have a significant impact on symptom management, emotional well-being, and overall quality of life.

Can I still exercise with gastroparesis?

I highly encourage most all GPers to incorporate exercise into their daily routine. Mild to moderate physical activity, such as walking, is often one of the most effective symptom management tools we have. Exercise can enhance gastric emptying, alleviate fullness, reduce bloating, improve bowel regularity, and relieve abdominal pain. It's also important for overall health, reducing blood pressure, increasing immunity, improving sleep, alleviating anxiety, and reducing the risk of heart disease and diabetes.

Aim for at least 30 minutes of physical activity each day. You may find that doing several shorter periods of activity throughout the day (before or after meals, for example) works best for symptom management. If you're currently sedentary, start small—take just a 10–15 minute walk after dinner, for example. Again, some is better than none!

What types of exercise are best?

When exercising to manage gastroparesis, the key is intensity. If you work out too hard, you'll likely experience *increased* symptoms. In fact, studies have shown that moderate physical activity causes the stomach to empty more quickly, but strenuous activity actually delays gastric emptying. (That's why even a healthy person may feel sick to their stomach during an intense workout.)

Longer, slower exercise is typically the most helpful and well tolerated for those with gastroparesis. I'm partial to walking, since it's free, easy, and versatile. You can walk outside, on a treadmill, or even in your living room with in-home walking DVDs. You can vary the intensity based on how you're feeling on any given day, and it's an activity that friends or family members can join you in doing.

Yoga is another excellent form of exercise for GPers and is equally versatile, ranging from gentle and restorative to athletic and physically challenging. Yoga may be especially beneficial for gastroparesis management, due to the integration of physical activity and stress reduction. If you're new to yoga, start with a yoga class led by an experienced teacher to learn which postures and sequences are best for you. Once you're familiar with the basics of yoga, you may choose to practice at home with the help of books or DVDs. A regular yoga practice can be an important part of a GP-management plan.

Of course there are a variety of other options, from biking to swimming to aerobics, and you should choose whichever is most enjoyable and comfortable for you. If you notice increased symptoms, take the intensity down and/or try a different activity.

Will exercise cause me to lose more weight?

Exercising in a way that's consistent with gastroparesis management may actually help with weight maintenance. Since physical activity reduces overall symptoms and often stimulates the appetite, it may allow you to eat more throughout the day. The extra calories that you're able to take in will likely meet or exceed those you'll burn via mild to moderate exercise.

Personally, I've found that I lose weight when I do not exercise regularly. Daily physical activity, specifically walking and yoga, has helped me to maintain the ten pounds I gained following my gastric neurostimulator surgery two years ago. Many of my clients have had similar experiences.

Does that mean I shouldn't exercise if I'm trying to lose weight?

Physical activity is important for health and well-being, whether or not it leads to weight loss. By reducing the symptoms associated with GP, exercise may allow you to better balance your diet and better nourish your body, thereby facilitating weight loss. What's more, regular physical activity helps to decrease stress and enhance sleep, both of which are important for intentional weight loss.

I'm already fatigued. Won't exercise just make it worse?

Regular physical activity can actually improve energy levels. Studies have shown that consistent exercise reduces fatigue, even among those with chronic medical conditions. It also promotes better sleep and is likely to boost your energy level throughout the day. Try starting with just 10–15 minutes of gentle activity during the time of day when you're least fatigued. Work up to 30 minutes or more as you're able.

Why are my symptoms worse when I don't sleep well?

The average adult needs seven to nine hours of sleep per night. Getting less than that can affect your energy level, mood, and metabolism. It can also affect your digestion. In fact, studies have shown that many patients with functional gastrointestinal disorders experience increased symptoms the morning after a restless night. In part that's because digestion, absorption, and assimilation of food is a process that requires a great deal of energy. Adequate, restful sleep ensures that your digestive organs, as well as the autonomic nervous system which controls the digestive process, have time for rest and repair.

Lack of sleep makes you more susceptible to stress, which can significantly influence digestive symptoms. What's more, daytime fatigue may lead to cravings for sugar or increase your overall appetite, causing you to eat more or differently than you normally would to manage symptoms.

Is it okay to have a snack before bed?   *important for me*

While some people find that their symptoms are best controlled by not eating between dinner and bedtime, others notice that a small snack shortly before bed actually improves sleep by preventing low blood sugar during the night. Nocturnal hypoglycemia can occur if your stomach empties all at once during the night, causing a rush of insulin that pushes blood sugar too low. You may wake up for seemingly no reason, or you might feel shaky, dizzy, or agitated.

A GP-friendly snack two to three hours before bed can prevent nocturnal hypoglycemia. The snack should contain both carbohydrates and protein. That's because protein contains an amino acid called tryptophan, which helps to make you sleepy, and the brain needs carbohydrates in order to utilize that tryptophan. Good choices include a piece of toast with a tablespoon of nut butter, a bowl of cereal with soy or skim milk, or crackers with an ounce of reduced-fat cheese.

Live Well Tip: Sleep Better

If you're having trouble sleeping, the following diet and lifestyle changes may help.

- Limit caffeine consumption, especially after noon. Caffeine is a stimulant that works by blocking the action of hormones in the brain that makes you feel sleepy. Caffeine can remain in the body for up to 12 hours.

- Avoid nicotine, especially at night.

- Avoid alcohol, especially in the evening. Alcohol may help you to relax and fall asleep, but it can disrupt sleep over the course of the night and decrease the overall quality of sleep.

- Practice relaxation techniques, such as deep abdominal breathing or progressive muscle relaxation, after getting into bed.

- Reduce digestive discomfort by sleeping on your left side (consider getting a wedge or body pillow).

- Elevate your head by 6 to 9 inches to alleviate reflux symptoms, either with a wedge between your box spring and mattress or by using risers on the head of the bed.

- Establish a regular, relaxing bedtime routine that will allow you to unwind and "signal" the brain that it's time to sleep. Avoid using the computer, smart phones, video games, etc. right before bed since they stimulate the brain.

- If you can't get to sleep after 30 minutes, get out of bed and do something relaxing, like reading a book. Try again when you feel sleepy.

- Chamomile tea offers a mild sedative effect, reducing anxiety and promoting sleep. It has also been shown to reduce nausea and indigestion. <u>Note: those with ragweed allergies should not consume chamomile.</u>

Does smoking affect gastroparesis?

Nicotine delays gastric emptying, so people with gastroparesis should not smoke. In addition, smoking decreases the strength of the lower esophageal sphincter, allowing stomach contents to reflux into the esophagus. This can exacerbate heartburn and regurgitation. Smoking can also increase the risk of other gastrointestinal problems, such as Crohn's disease, gallbladder diseases, and liver damage.

Can I drink alcohol?

Alcohol slows digestion of meals, especially those containing fat. Alcohol also impairs the quality of sleep, weakens the lower esophageal sphincter allowing contents of the stomach to reflux into the esophagus, can cause gastritis (inflammation of the lining of the stomach), and decreases the secretion of digestive enzymes from the pancreas. While some GPers are able to drink small amounts of alcohol from time to time, most find that avoiding alcohol is helpful for symptom management.

Does stress cause gastroparesis?

Stress doesn't cause gastroparesis, but stress and digestion *are* very closely intertwined. Stress triggers what's known as the "fight or flight" response or the stress response. This is an evolutionary process designed to keep us alive in dangerous situations.

In order to prepare the body to run or fight, the stress response activates the sympathetic nervous system and releases stress hormones like adrenaline and cortisol. Heart rate, blood sugar, and blood pressure increase and the body shuts down all processes that are not essential for survival—including digestion. After the immediate stressor is eliminated, your hormone levels drop and your regular body functions resume.

Unfortunately, many of us are constantly stressed, and the body can't differentiate life-or-death stress from the stress caused by family, jobs, or chronic illness. This means we're constantly activating the stress response and, as I mentioned, part of the stress response is to shut down non-essential processes like digestion. This is why chronic stress can exacerbate gastroparesis symptoms and make the other parts of your management plan less effective.

Live Well Tip: Get to Know Your Second Brain

The enteric nervous system (ENS) is the nervous system within the gut. It's sometimes called the "second brain." The role of the ENS is to manage every aspect of digestion and regulate the function of the esophagus, stomach, small intestine, and colon.

The ENS is extremely complex. In fact, there are more nerve cells in the enteric nervous system than in the entire spinal cord. The ENS exchanges messages with the central nervous system via the vagus nerve. About 90 percent of those messages travel *from the gut to the brain*, not the other way around. In fact, animal studies have shown that the ENS can continue to regulate digestion on its own, even if the vagus nerve is severed.

The ENS utilizes over thirty neurotransmitters—many of the same ones used by the brain. For example, at least 90 percent of the body's serotonin, the "feel good" chemical, is made and stored in the gut. Serotonin plays a significant role in both digestion and mood, which is why antidepressants are often prescribed in the treatment of gastroparesis.

The study of the enteric nervous system (called neurogastroenterology) is a relatively new field. Researchers are just beginning to put the pieces together when it comes to the complicated ways the brain and the gut interact, as well as how the ENS functions and what causes it to malfunction. As more is discovered, treatment for FGIMDs such as gastroparesis will certainly improve.

For more information about the enteric nervous system, read *The Second Brain: A Groundbreaking New Understanding of Nervous Disorders of the Stomach and Intestine* by Michael Gershon, M.D.

Having gastroparesis is the most stressful part of my life. What do I do about that?

Stress comes from a variety of sources. Some stress is external; it can be caused by our families, job, or finances. Other stress is internal; it can be a result of our worries, beliefs, and thoughts. But the biggest source of stress for most people with gastroparesis is the gastroparesis itself. Michael Gershon captured this perfectly in the preface to his book *The Second Brain* when he wrote, "few things are more distressing than an inefficient gut with feeling."

While all chronic illnesses are stressful, digestive conditions like gastroparesis present a double whammy. That's because the gut is connected to the brain via bidirectional pathways. Messages go both ways: from the brain to the gut and from the gut to the brain. So while mental stress can trigger digestive distress, digestive distress can also cause mental stress.

The good news is that I know, from both personal and professional experience, that the better you manage your gastroparesis, the less stressful it becomes. Developing and following a comprehensive management plan based on the information in this book will make things a lot easier.

In my experience, the majority of GPers are people with type A personalities whose minds never stop going. Relaxation can be both difficult and uncomfortable, but it's probably what many of us need most. In fact, to counteract the "flight or fight" response, we must activate the relaxation response. This is a concept that was originally pioneered by a Dr. Herbert Benson. The idea is to use mindfulness and relaxation practices to calm the nervous system so that it stops releasing stress chemicals like cortisol and adrenaline. While activating the relaxation response probably won't cure your digestive troubles, it can certainly help to alleviate and manage symptoms over time.

I have trouble relaxing. How can I elicit the relaxation response?

There are a number of ways to evoke the relaxation response, including repetitive prayer, mindfulness meditations, relaxation exercises, and repetitive physical exercise, such as yoga or Tai Chi. Try a variety of things until you find the one that best suits you.

You may be uncomfortable with relaxation or find it difficult at first. The more you practice, the easier it will become. Schedule a time to practice every day and try to be consistent so that it becomes a natural part of your daily routine. Avoid practicing when you're sleepy. Find a time when you're awake, alert, and unlikely to be interrupted.

Aim for 10 to 20 minutes once or twice a day. As always, I encourage you to start small and build up. At first, a five-minute practice once a day may be easier to fit into your schedule. You'll still reap great benefits. Don't beat yourself up if you miss a day or even a few days. Just stick with it. These practices can be one of the most important parts of a gastroparesis management plan. For more information, read *The Relaxation Response* by Dr. Herbert Benson.

What should I do if I can't seem to manage the stress on my own?

If you are overwhelmed by stress or if you're struggling with depression or anxiety, seek help from a qualified mental health professional. Stress issues are common among people with chronic illness, especially people with FGIMDs, and there is absolutely no shame in obtaining treatment. It doesn't mean that your symptoms are in your head or that you're causing or exacerbating the illness. But because the brain and the gut are so intimately connected, better management of mental health issues is likely to lead to an improvement in your ability to manage your GP symptoms, as well as contribute to a better quality of life.

Live Well Tip: Learn to Manage GP-Related Stress

- **Be Flexible:** While there's much that you can do to alleviate your symptoms, there is a level of uncertainty that comes along with gastroparesis. The more flexible you can be, the less stressful the unpredictability will be.

- **Be Prepared:** Always be prepared with GP-friendly food and symptom management remedies. This makes being flexible much easier!

- **Give Yourself a Break:** Despite your best efforts, you're going to have bad days—emotionally and physically. It's normal. Beating yourself up on these days will only increase your internal stress. Instead, care for yourself as you would a sick child: with kindness and patience.

- **Focus on the Can-Do:** Concentrating your attention on the things that you can't do because of gastroparesis will only increase feelings of dissatisfaction. Make it a point to focus on what you can do...and do it! Find a new hobby or reengage in an old one. Find something that you enjoy doing that fits into your life with gastroparesis. crochet

- Avoid Self-Pity: An occasional "why me?" moment is to be expected, but ongoing pity parties just aren't a good use of your time or energy. Feeling like you don't have control of a situation is often what makes it stressful. So identify your challenges, and then find constructive ways to deal with them. *doctors labs tests*

- Respect Your Limitations: Pushing yourself beyond your limits, whether that means eating something you shouldn't or not getting proper rest, is a sure-fire way to exacerbate your symptoms. Learn to say no. Learn to delegate. Cut yourself some slack.

- Take Good Care of Yourself: Put your gastroparesis management plan into place and be consistent in the choices you make. Nourish your body and your mind. If you're sleep-deprived, malnourished, or highly symptomatic, it's much more difficult to manage stress.

- Ask Questions: Many of the fears and anxieties that we feel, especially those related to gastroparesis, are due to uncertainty and what-ifs. When you have the knowledge that comes from getting your questions answered, it often puts your mind at ease. Call upon the members of your Dream Team to address any questions or concerns you have.

- Help Others: Sometimes the best way to take your mind off your own worries is to help someone else. Volunteer for a cause that is important to you or practice random acts of kindness.

LIFE WITH GASTROPARESIS

What you do every day matters more than what you do once in a while.

–Gretchen Rubin

Educating yourself about the various aspects of gastroparesis management is important, but it's not very useful if you can't incorporate those things into your everyday life. Remember, your whole life needs to be GP-friendly—not just your diet or your personal habits. This means figuring out how to handle things like relationships, socializing, working, and traveling. Once these things fall into place, living *well* with gastroparesis requires less effort on an ongoing basis.

How do I help my family and friends understand what I'm going through?

The first thing to realize is that we can't expect people to understand something they know nothing about. Those of us who live with gastroparesis day in and day out may forget that most other people have never heard of the condition. In order for your family and friends to understand what you're going through, you have to educate them.

When explaining gastroparesis to others, try to make it relatable and concise. Rather than using words like "motility disorder," for example, say something like, "I have a digestive condition called gastroparesis. That means my stomach doesn't empty food as quickly as it should. It's kind of like having the stomach flu all the time." Most people have had the stomach flu and can relate to the nausea, vomiting, and fatigue that come along with it.

Don't forget to explain your new limitations and priorities so that your family and friends understand why what they're seeing from you now might be different from what they are used to. It's important to point out that you have good days and bad days, and that the condition tends to be unpredictable. Let people know up front that you may have to cancel or change plans in order to accommodate your symptoms on any given day. By making this clear in advance, it can help to prevent misunderstandings, judgments, and hurt feelings.

You may also wish to explain that gastroparesis is an invisible illness. You may look quite healthy, even when you are feeling very sick. You can also point out that you're more likely to be social and seen out-and-about on your good days, when your symptoms aren't as severe.

For many people, especially acquaintances or distant family, that will be enough. Others will be genuinely interested and may ask follow-up questions. In these cases you can offer to share resources with them, such as this book or informational websites. With close family members, you may even want to invite them to attend doctor's appointments so that they can learn more and ask questions.

I don't want my family and friends to treat me like a sick person. Should I just keep quiet?

If you don't want others to feel sorry for you or treat you like a "sick person," then you have to set that example in the way that you talk about the condition and approach your life with gastroparesis. When you're educating your family and friends, for example, avoid phrases like "suffering from" in favor of more proactive words like "managing." It's also important to keep your sense of self, remembering that gastroparesis is a part of your life—but it doesn't have to be your whole life. If you set that example, others will follow suit.

How can I deal with loved ones who aren't always supportive?

Aside from helping the people in your life understand the condition, you also have to let them know the ways in which they can best support you. They may not know what to do to help you feel better physically or to support you emotionally. Ask for what you need and you're far more likely to get it.

Also be sure to acknowledge the ways in which your loved ones themselves are affected by the situation. Show them the kind of support and patience that you are expecting in return. They may feel helpless, scared, or even angry. Letting them know that you understand that they are also facing new challenges due to the gastroparesis can go a long way.

Even after you've made a proper attempt to educate the people in your life about gastroparesis and the type of support you need, there are some who just will not get it. In these cases you either have to accept that fact and deal with it or choose to distance yourself from the person. Either way, continue to stand up for your needs and respect your limitations.

How do I explain this to my children?

It's important to explain gastroparesis to children in an age-appropriate manner and frame it in a way that they can understand, whether that means "mom doesn't feel well" or "mommy has a tummy ache." A good resource on this topic is *Raising an Emotionally Healthy Child When a Parent is Sick* (A Harvard Medical School Book) by Paula Rausch, MD.

How should I handle comments about my weight or my food choices?

When people make offensive comments about your food choices or your appearance, they may be concerned, genuinely curious, or even jealous. Depending on the motivation and your relationship to someone, you can either choose to let it go or speak up. If you don't see the person often, it might be just as easy to ignore the comment. However, if it's a friend, family member, or co-worker, it's best to address the situation in order to prevent similar comments in the future.

Explain nicely that you appreciate the concern; however, your dietary choices and weight fluctuations are directly related to your current health issues and you are doing the best you can to manage both. If a comment is especially ignorant or insensitive (for instance, if someone says that they wish they had GP so they too could lose weight), it's okay for you to express your feelings. Calmly explain that you find the comment hurtful because it minimizes the pain that the illness has caused you and emphasize that you wouldn't wish it on anyone for any reason. If someone continues to make offensive or inappropriate comments even after you have tried to educate them, you may need to reduce the amount of time you spend with that person.

Live Well Tip: Look Good, Feel Good

How you look affects the way you feel. That might sound trite, but I believe it's true. I've found that paying attention to my appearance, regardless of how I feel physically, boosts my mood and lifts my spirits.

over

I think some GPers are hesitant to look *too good* for fear that others might not recognize or believe that they're ill. But really, who cares? Why should you look like a mess just so people know you feel lousy? It won't make you feel any better. So even on my bad days—especially on my bad days—I put some effort into my appearance. I choose an outfit that's comfortable but pretty—something I feel good wearing. I put on nice earrings or cute shoes.

The key here is to have clothes that reflect your style, fit well, and are GP-friendly. If you've lost weight with gastroparesis, buy some new clothes. If you've gained weight, buy some new clothes. Look for clothes that have extra room in the stomach to accommodate bloating or a painful abdomen. Empire-waist tops and dresses, for example, or stretchy leggings that can be worn with tunics or long sweaters. Maternity clothes are actually fantastic for hiding a bloated belly and there are lots of stylish, affordable options at stores like Target and Old Navy.

How can I maintain my friendships?

Maintaining friendships can be one of the most difficult aspects of living with gastroparesis. Feeling as if others don't understand, many GPers find themselves becoming more and more socially isolated as time goes on. Rather than distance yourself during this challenging time, make an effort to reach out to your friends. They may be unsure about the best way to support you, so go ahead and tell them. Support comes in many forms, and it might vary based on the relationship. Certain friends may provide a shoulder to lean on, while others may offer a distraction from your pain and worries. *Dave* *Joy*

Here are some GP-friendly ways to connect with your friends:

- Schedule regular phone calls.

- Meet for coffee or tea.

- Go for a walk together.

- Talk about non-GP-related things.

- Learn to cook GP-friendly recipes together.

- Join a yoga class together.

- Join or start a book club together.

The stronger your relationships, the better off you'll be as you navigate life with gastroparesis. Loneliness makes everything more daunting. Of course, not all relationships are strong enough to withstand something like chronic illness. Superficial friendships are likely to fall by the wayside. One of the benefits of GP is that you will truly learn who your friends are. Just remember that half the work of keeping up friendships is still yours.

How do I continue being social if I can't eat or drink normally?

Covid

Socializing can be difficult for GPers since most social activities tend to revolve around eating and drinking. Very rarely does someone ask you to do something that doesn't involve some kind of consumption. While going to food-centered places and events can be uncomfortable, sometimes it's unavoidable and you just have to make the best of it. Other times, however, you can (and should!) steer the activity toward something more GP-friendly.

Here are some ideas:

- Movies

- Miniature golf

- Bowling

- Concerts

- Festivals

- Game nights

- Sporting events

- Antiquing

- Shopping

- Bingo

- Museums

- Plays

- Outdoor activities like hiking or biking

Of course, another obstacle to being social is not feeling well. Constant nausea, a bloated belly, or stomach pain don't make for a comfortable night out. However, you may notice that when you're just feeling slightly ill, getting out and having some fun can actually distract you from your symptoms. If you're really feeling lousy, consider inviting a friend over to watch a movie or chat. Sometimes you'll just want to lie down or be by yourself, but try to avoid isolating yourself every time you don't feel well.

How do I handle advice from people who don't know anything about GP?

Most of the time when people offer advice, they're trying to be helpful. Because gastroparesis is not a widely-known condition, it's likely that the advice offered may not be appropriate. Simply thank the person for the concern and either say that you'll look into it further or explain that you already have a comprehensive management plan that is working well for you.

If, however, what they say interests you, research it thoroughly and talk with the members of your Dream Team to ensure that the advice is safe and suitable for your situation.

Live Well Tip: Eating Out with Gastroparesis

The key to successfully dining out with gastroparesis is preparation. Try to make plans in advance and do your homework prior to mealtime. While this takes the spontaneity out of going out to eat, it usually makes the experience more enjoyable and less stressful.

Here are some tips:

Speak up. If possible, suggest a restaurant that you know will have something on the menu that you can eat, or at least try to nix options that you know will not have GP-friendly choices. Mexican restaurants, for example, typically offer little that GPers can eat without a great deal of modification. Seafood restaurants, on the other hand, usually have several options.

Research the menu. Once you know where you're going, especially if it wasn't your choice, try to research the menu. Almost all chain restaurants and many independent establishments post their menus online. Some also provide nutrition information, which is extremely valuable, since seemingly healthy dishes can sometimes be surprisingly high in fat. You can also call ahead to find out what the soup selections or other specials are for that day.

Decide what to order in advance. One of the most stressful parts of going out to eat is deciding what to order. You want something that is least likely to cause symptoms—especially if you have plans after dinner—but you also want to enjoy your meal. It can also be uncomfortable to look over the menu as the others in your party look on, asking if there's anything you can eat or suggesting things that they think you should be able to eat. If possible, decide what you'll order before you arrive. That way you won't even have to open the menu!

Have a Plan B. There's nothing worse than being hungry and finding there's nothing on the menu that you can or want to eat. Always have your own stash of GP-friendly items that can you pull out in a pinch.

Enjoy the company. Regardless of how things turn out food-wise, do your best to focus your attention on the people that you're with and enjoy the company and conversation. Being social and continuing to spend time with friends—even if that means just watching other people eat once in a while—is usually better for the spirit than sitting at home alone!

For special occasions...

When you're going out to eat for a special occasion (like a birthday, graduation, or anniversary) you may wish to call the restaurant in advance to discuss meal options. Tell them when you will be dining at the restaurant and explain that you have dietary restrictions due to a medical condition. They'll often let you talk directly to the chef and, more often than not, the chef will be willing to work with you to modify an existing dish so that it's GP-friendly or even come up with a special meal just for you. By arranging everything ahead of time, you won't have to ask questions or make special requests on the spot and you'll be able to enjoy the celebratory meal with your family and friends.

How do I handle invitations to dinner parties?

While it's easy to plan ahead when going to a restaurant, meals at other people's homes can be more difficult to navigate since there are personal feelings involved. It's best to be up front with the host or hostess about the fact that you have dietary restrictions. Emphasize that what you're really looking forward to is their company.

Some people may ask if they can prepare special food for you, but it's usually best to just bring food that you know you can eat. People who don't have any experience with GP often don't know or understand the complexities of the dietary restrictions or your personal tolerances. Depending on the situation and your comfort level, you can either make yourself a plate of GP-friendly food to be served with everyone else's meal or bring a GP-friendly dish that you can eat and share with others.

What should I do at special events, like weddings or holiday parties, which include a served meal?

If you've been invited to a special celebration and you know the host or hostess well, consider contacting them to discuss your dietary restrictions. Often times they'll be able to request a special meal for you. Be specific about what you can and cannot eat, and offer suggestions based on the meals offered. This will allow you to fully participate in the event, hopefully without exacerbating symptoms.

If you don't feel comfortable discussing your needs, select the meal option that most closely resembles something you know you can tolerate and eat just a small amount. Of course you can always choose to forgo the meal entirely, making sure to eat a GP-friendly meal before you arrive. Either way, be sure that you have medication or other remedies on-hand in case symptoms do occur.

How can I date when I have gastroparesis?

Dating when you have any chronic illness is difficult, but gastroparesis presents an additional obstacle, since it's difficult to meet for drinks or go out to dinner. When you meet someone new, it's important to be up front about the fact that you have gastroparesis. Don't dwell on it, however. Briefly explain the condition and then move on. Your date wants to get to know you, and you are about so much more than gastroparesis.

In terms of choosing date activities, offer suggestions that don't revolve around food or involve only food that you know you can tolerate. Dating is stressful enough without worrying about gastroparesis. If your potential date doesn't understand this, isn't flexible, or seems annoyed, he or she is not the right fit for you anyway.

Can people with gastroparesis get pregnant and have healthy babies?

Many women have become pregnant and given birth to healthy babies despite having gastroparesis. Unfortunately, there has been little research done and few resources available specifically for moms-to-be with GP, so an attentive, knowledgeable doctor is extremely important. Women should focus on obtaining adequate nutrition, both from diet and supplementation. If additional nutrition is necessary, temporary artificial nutrition is an option.

Many of the medications used to enhance gastric emptying and/or to treat the symptoms of gastroparesis may not be safe for use during pregnancy, so alternative methods of symptom management become even more important at that time. Physical activity, stress management, relaxation practices, dietary modifications, and certain complementary therapies can help to alleviate both the symptoms of GP and of pregnancy, such as nausea, heartburn, and constipation.

If you plan to become pregnant, talk with your health care providers about these things in advance. As with nearly everything else involving gastroparesis, adequate preparation will likely lead to a better outcome.

How do I maintain my job after I've been diagnosed with gastroparesis?

Though I'm not an expert in this field, my advice is to be honest and up front with your employer. Explain the diagnosis and how it might affect your ability to perform your work. You may need certain accommodations in order to manage your symptoms, such as four 15-minute breaks rather than a one-hour lunch. If your job is especially stressful or the schedule is inflexible, you may need to inquire about other positions within the company or even explore other options.

Most people with gastroparesis are able to continue working, whether in their original position or in one more conducive to symptom management. If, however, your symptoms prevent you from being able to work altogether, you may apply for Social Security Disability Insurance. Keep in mind that it's a lengthy process; you have to prove that you cannot work in any capacity, and compensation is quite small.

If at some point you find yourself unable to work or if you're working less than you're used to, try to find a constructive way to use your skills and free time. Whether that means taking up a new hobby or volunteering for a cause you're passionate about, doing something to take your mind off of your symptoms and give a purpose to your days is important for morale.

Can I still travel with gastroparesis?

While traveling with gastroparesis presents a number of challenges, it can be done successfully and enjoyably. The key is proper planning and continued adherence to your management plan.

While on vacation continue to follow your regular schedule, both in terms of diet and lifestyle activities, as closely as possible. For example, if you typically practice yoga or relaxation exercises in the morning, be sure to include those in your daily itinerary.

While eating away from home, continue to focus on maximizing nutrition in every bite and sip you take. This is not the time to consume "empty" foods that fill you up without providing any nutrients. Without proper nutrition, you're less likely to have the energy to fully enjoy your vacation.

If you choose to experiment, do so carefully and deliberately. If you're going to try something you wouldn't ordinarily eat at home, don't do it impulsively. Be sure you have the time and flexibility to relax afterward should you feel sick. Always respect your limitations and allow yourself to rest if you feel tired or symptomatic.

Continue to be active, especially after meals. Many people find that walking helps to alleviate symptoms and improve digestion. It's also a great way to explore your vacation destination! But be sure to drink plenty of water, especially if you're traveling by air, vacationing somewhere warm, and/or engaging in physical activity. In addition to causing headaches and dizziness, dehydration can exacerbate symptoms of nausea and vomiting.

The point of vacation is to have fun, so find ways to indulge that do not include food, such as treating yourself to a spa service or a special activity with your friends or family. While the demands of managing gastroparesis can seem overwhelming, especially on vacation, adhering to these tips will allow you to more fully enjoy your time away.

Live Well Tip: Traveling With Gastroparesis

While managing gastroparesis at home can be difficult, traveling poses an even greater challenge. With the right preparation, however, it *is* possible to enjoy time away with family and friends without compromising symptom management.

Before You Go

- Be sure to take your needs into account when making travel arrangements.

  o If you'll be staying in a hotel, request a room with a small refrigerator or kitchenette. This gives you the flexibility to store and/or prepare some of your own food.

  o If you'll be staying with friends or family, inform them of your medical condition and consequent dietary restrictions. Either provide a detailed list of what you can and cannot eat or let them know that you will be bringing and preparing your own food.

  o If you'll be traveling by air and will need to bring liquid meal replacements or medication on board your flight, contact the TSA at 1-866-289-9673 to make special arrangements. If you have the Enterra gastric neurostimulator, be sure to pack the device identification card in your carry-on luggage so that you can present it at all security check points.

- Keep an ongoing list of gastroparesis-friendly foods that you know you can eat safely. This will come in handy when dining away from home.

- Pack nutrient-dense, portable snacks for travel days and an ample amount of gastroparesis-friendly staples for the duration of your trip.

- Pack all medications, supplements, remedies, and symptom management tools that you use at home (whether on a regular or an as-needed or emergency basis).

- If you rely on smoothies, purees, or protein shakes as part of your daily diet, invest in a portable blender (such as a Magic Bullet) to use when you reach your destination.

Travel Day

- Regardless of how you're traveling, bring your own food and pack twice as much you think you'll need. Delays are unpredictable, and you can never be sure there will be gastroparesis-friendly options along the way.

- You may find that you're more prone to motion sickness than you were prior to having gastroparesis. Have a variety of nausea remedies on hand, just in case. I always carry a QueaseEASE when traveling (www.soothing-scents.com).

- Follow your typical meal plan as closely as possible. Rather than snacking all day, which is likely to provide little nutrition and leave you feeling full but unsatisfied, eat well-balanced mini-meals at regular intervals.

- Eat mindfully and in a relaxed environment—not in the car or while walking through the airport. Take a few breaths to relax before you start eating, and chew your food thoroughly to help facilitate digestion.

COPING & ATTITUDE

To get through the hardest journey we need take only one step at a time, but we must keep on stepping.

–Chinese proverb

The emotional challenges of living with gastroparesis are often just as great as the physical ones. Yet learning to cope is absolutely imperative for managing your symptoms and improving your quality of life. Coming to terms with the condition is a process and it's normal to feel frustrated, confused, sad, or angry from time to time. The key to living well with gastroparesis is to not waste valuable time and energy wallowing in those feelings. Instead, figure out the best course of action and face the challenges head on.

How do I begin to effectively cope with gastroparesis?

In my opinion the first step to being able to cope with gastroparesis is accepting that you have gastroparesis. That might sound odd; after all, you bought a book about living with gastroparesis. Clearly you accept that you have the condition, right? Not necessarily. There's a difference between acknowledgment and acceptance, and while it's easy to acknowledge that we have the condition, it's much more difficult to accept that fact.

If you find yourself ruminating over how unfair it is that you have gastroparesis or fixating on how much better things would be if you didn't have gastroparesis, that's not acceptance. If you find yourself purposefully doing things that you know will cause your symptoms to flare up in an act of rebellion against the condition, that's not acceptance. Besides being mentally exhausting, a fight against reality is one you'll never win. And when you're spending so much energy resisting the fact that you have gastroparesis, it's difficult to manage the condition and nearly impossible to *live well* with it.

It's important to understand that acceptance doesn't mean that you're happy about the situation. It also doesn't mean giving up hope that things will improve. Accepting that you have gastroparesis today does not mean that you're going to have gastroparesis next week, next month, or next year. It's about accepting your current reality so that you can take effective action to improve your wellbeing and quality of life for the future.

What if I'm just angry and feel like I can't accept this?

Finding acceptance doesn't happen overnight. There is an adjustment period between diagnosis and acceptance, the length of which varies from person to person. It's important to give yourself the necessary time and space to go through the process and come to terms with your new reality.

You should expect an ebb and flow in your emotions, just as you expect an ebb and flow in your physical symptoms. Not every day is a good day. Seven-plus years after my diagnosis, I still have days where I can't find acceptance or patience. Fortunately, those days are much less frequent than they were a few years ago. It gets easier, especially as you educate yourself and learn to better manage your physical symptoms.

Trust in the fact that your bad days will give way to good days, just as your physical flare-ups eventually pass. On your bad days, treat yourself with extra kindness and compassion. It's not a direct path from diagnosis to acceptance or from education to living well, and there's really no end point. It's a process, and there will be ups and downs.

I feel like my whole life revolves around gastroparesis now. Is that normal?

It's common to become consumed with gastroparesis, especially right after diagnosis or during flare ups. Between trying to understand the condition and trying to manage the symptoms, you may find that it's all you think about. (If you're not sure whether it's consuming you, ask your family what you talk about most often. If they instantly yell out, "Gastroparesis!" that's a good clue.)

Putting *all* of your focus on gastroparesis isn't healthy, and it isn't necessary in order to live well with the condition. You have not become "Gastroparesis." You are still you, a person with a family, interests, and a life outside of the condition. Having gastroparesis may affect the choices that you make (it should if you're following a management plan), but it doesn't have to be the center of your universe.

Being consumed with thoughts of gastroparesis, even if your intention is to be proactive, is exhausting. While you're learning to manage GP, don't let go of the other parts of your life.

Continue going to your book club, making art, or playing with your kids—whatever brings you joy, lets you decompress, and reminds you that gastroparesis is not your whole life. This alone can improve your attitude, energy level, and quality of life. (You'll also have an easier time connecting with family and friends if you have something to talk about other than gastroparesis!)

I feel like I don't have any control over my symptoms. How can I accept the uncertainty?

You're not responsible for having gastroparesis, but you are responsible for how you choose to deal with it. And while it might seem like you have very little control over how you feel day to day, you have quite a bit more than you think. It's up to you, for example, whether you prioritize self-care. It's up to you to be proactive when it comes to managing your Dream Team. It's up to you to choose the most nutrient-rich foods that your symptoms allow and to take your vitamins regularly.

Does that mean you have *complete* control? Sadly, no. Gastroparesis symptoms may flare up for reasons that you can do nothing about—monthly hormone cycles, for example, or triggers you can't even identify. But how well you implement the suggestions outlined in this book (and the choices that you make every day) will directly influence how you feel much of the time.

I've had so many clients tell me in their first session, "It doesn't matter what I do; I feel sick every day." A few sessions later, this inevitably switches to, "I never realized how much control I have over how I feel on a daily basis." I can almost guarantee that if you put together a comprehensive management plan that addresses each of the areas we've discussed in this book, you will find yourself in a better place physically and mentally.

How do I get over the fear that comes with having GP?

Those with gastroparesis are often consumed with fear. Fear of eating, fear of flare-ups, fear of never getting better, fear of socializing, fear of traveling, fear of not being taken seriously…the list goes on. Ironically, it's often the fear—not the condition—that keeps many GPers trapped within the confines of malnutrition, exhaustion, illness and/or loneliness.

Acknowledge the ways in which your GP-related fears are holding you back from better managing your symptoms, improving your overall health, or leading a more fulfilling life…

and then do something about it. Are you afraid to vary your diet because you might get sick? Try one new GP-friendly food this week. Are you afraid to exercise because you might feel worse? Take a walk around the block after dinner and see what happens. Afraid to try a new treatment because it might not work? Consider the implications of not trying. Afraid to put your needs first because others might think you're lazy or selfish? Make self-care your top priority for *one day* and see how you feel.

I'm certainly not encouraging you to be reckless. It's not about eating or doing things that you know aren't good for you. It's about stepping outside of your comfort zone in order to acknowledge and address the fears that are keeping you from a happier, healthier life. While you must always respect your limitations and make smart choices, you might be surprised just how much your world opens up once you let go of the fear.

How do I find the time and money for all of this self-care?

What's the one thing in your life that, if it changed, would change everything else? Whatever your answer is, you have to make that thing a priority and invest your time, money, and energy accordingly. If that thing happens to be better gastroparesis management, then I assure you that self-care is essential.

That might mean you have to cut yourself some slack in other areas or learn to delegate responsibilities at work or home. But when we don't put self-care first, we're not only doing ourselves a disservice, we're doing our families and the other people who count on us a disservice, as well. The better you can manage your physical symptoms and emotional stress, the better spouse, parent, child, sibling, friend, and employee you will be. Guaranteed.

Start paying more attention to your actions. Do they reflect your priorities? If you want to live well with gastroparesis, you must take a hard look at the choices you're making every day and ensure that they match up with that goal.

Where can I find support?

Support is a very important part of coping with gastroparesis. People who feel isolated or lonely are typically less able to cope with the ups and downs of any chronic illness. Building a strong support system is similar in some ways to building your Dream Team. You have to put together a team of people who uplift you and empower you to live well. Your support system may include family members, friends, mental health practitioners, or other GPers whom you've connected with in person or online. The important thing is that people in your support system help you to focus on the ways in which you can address the challenges you're facing, not just dwell on the challenges themselves.

Avoid people who make you feel worse about your situation, whether by challenging the validity of your symptoms, encouraging you to behave in ways that do not correspond with proper management, or engaging you in competitive suffering. If you're not sure if certain people or groups are appropriate members of your support system, think about how they make you feel. Empowered? Optimistic? Depressed? Hopeless? Good support lifts you up. It doesn't drag you down.

Is there any hope that my gastroparesis will improve over time?

Very little is currently known about FGIMDs in general and gastroparesis in particular (especially idiopathic gastroparesis). While that may sound like bad news to some, it actually represents a tremendous opportunity. It means that each new discovery is likely to bring about advancements in treatment options. If we knew all there was to know about gastroparesis and yet there was no medical cure, now that would be a pretty hopeless situation. Luckily, that's not the case. There are physicians and researchers who are dedicating their careers to studying the enteric nervous system and functional GI motility disorders. Breakthroughs and better treatment for those of us with gastroparesis are imminent.

What's more, GP is a dynamic condition. It doesn't often stay the same from month to month or year to year. I've worked with many people who have gotten better over time. A comprehensive management plan, like the one we've talked about throughout this book, can make a big difference in your ability to live well with gastroparesis or even eventually *get well*.

Is there anything I can do to ensure that better treatments are found?

The major roadblock to a better understanding of gastroparesis is not lack of ability—it's lack of funding. And not only is funding necessary for research, adequate funding will be essential in order to translate scientific discoveries into practical applications that will affect the treatment that you and I receive. Currently, FGIMDs as a group, including gastroparesis, are disproportionately underfunded.

But it doesn't have to be that way. We can change it. Funding is political. It has nothing to do with the prevalence or severity of a condition. It comes down to how you and I educate our lawmakers about our needs as GPers and ask them to do something about it. The squeaky wheel gets the grease, right? To get involved in the advocacy effort, visit www.DHA.org or www.GPDFoundation.org.

Live Well Tip: Paint a Silver Lining

You can certainly approach gastroparesis as if nothing good can come out of it. After all, there's no inherent silver lining in not being able to eat normally. The good news is, we have the freedom to paint our own silver lining: to take this life-altering situation that we didn't ask for and ensure that it alters our life in the best way possible.

While your silver line may start out barely visible—you have a little more compassion for others or you made a new friend in your GP support group—the more you divert your focus from the muck in the middle to that silver lining around the edge, the thicker it gets. Does that mean the mess inside the cloud is any less dark? Not really. There's still physical pain and logistical challenges and emotional struggles. But when you have that pretty, shiny line around the outside, the mess in the middle is no longer your sole focus.

The difference between people who learn to live well with gastroparesis and those who don't, largely comes down to a willingness to paint a silver lining. Without that silver lining, you're left with nothing but doom and gloom You can take medication and get acupuncture and exercise regularly and sleep well…but you're still living underneath a dark cloud. You don't have to be happy or grateful to have gastroparesis in order to get out your paintbrush (I don't think anybody fits that description). You simply have to *want to live well with gastroparesis*.

Today my silver lining is thick and shiny. It's made up of blessings I'd never thought to wish for and growth I didn't know I was capable of. I'm incredibly grateful for my family—my mom, dad, brother and husband—who have been by my side (and on my side!) since the day I was diagnosed. I've proven to myself that I'm stronger mentally and physically than I ever imagined I could be. I feel truly blessed that you are reading these words and grateful that you have allowed me to be a part of your journey.

When I was diagnosed with gastroparesis in 2004, I never imagined that seven years later I'd be writing a book about the condition. Standing in that doctor's office, I never dreamed that I'd have the opportunity to touch so many lives and offer hope to people who feel as lost now as I felt that day. While I'm not thankful to have gastroparesis, I am thankful for my silver lining. I hope that this book helps you to find your own silver lining and live *well* with gastroparesis.

Recipes

Too much sugar

Too much potassium

Author's Note

I encourage you to think of these recipes as a starting point for experimentation. I've included a variety of options, from liquids to soft foods to GP-friendly versions of traditional dishes. Many are wheat free and/or milk free. But while all of these recipes can be considered GP-friendly, not all of them may be appropriate for you at this time. Likewise, the proper serving size for you may vary from what's listed.

You may need to tailor certain recipes to better suit your personal tolerances and/or preferences. For that reason, the nutritional information provided is only an *estimate*. The exact amount of fat and fiber per serving will vary based on the brand of ingredients that you use and the substitutions that you make.

Because many products contain traces of gluten or dairy, recipes are designated as "wheat free" or "milk free" rather than gluten free or dairy free. All such recipes can be prepared completely gluten free and/or dairy free depending on the brand of ingredients that you use.

Breakfast, Brunch & Breads

Never work before breakfast; if you have to work before breakfast, eat your breakfast first.

–Josh Billings

Old-Fashioned Pancakes

8 Servings

Who needs a pancake mix? This from-scratch recipe is easy to prepare and can be customized to your personal tolerances and preferences.

Ingredients

- 1-1/2 cups all-purpose flour

- 3-1/2 teaspoons baking powder

- 1/2 teaspoon salt

- 1 tablespoon maple syrup

- 1-1/4 cups dairy or non-dairy milk

- 1 egg

- 2 tablespoons butter, melted

Directions

Sift together flour, baking powder, and salt in a large bowl. Make a well in the center and pour in maple syrup, milk, egg, and melted butter. Stir until combined, but do not over mix. Heat a griddle over medium-high heat. Spray with nonstick cooking spray. Pour the batter by the ¼ cup onto hot griddle. Cook until bubbles appear on surface and then flip. Cook an additional 2–3 minutes on the other side. Serve with maple syrup, yogurt, or GPNB (see page 148).

Variation: top each pancake with sliced bananas or diced peaches and a sprinkling of cinnamon before flipping to the second side.

Approximately 3.5 grams of fat and 1 gram of fiber per serving.

Peanut Butter Banana Pancake for One

1 Serving

This one-serving pancake offers a good balance of protein, carbohydrates, and healthy fat to start your day, plus it features one of my favorite flavor combinations: peanut butter and bananas!

Ingredients

- 1/4 cup all-purpose flour

- 1/2 teaspoon baking powder

- 1 medium ripe banana

- 1 egg, lightly beaten

- 1/2 teaspoon vanilla extract

- 1 tablespoon GPNB (see page 148)

Directions

In a small bowl, combine flour and baking powder. In a separate bowl, mash banana, then add egg and vanilla. Stir the banana mixture into the dry ingredients just until moistened. Batter will be thick. Pour batter onto a hot griddle coated with cooking spray. Cook until bubbles form on the surface, then flip and cook until golden brown. Spread with GPNB.

Approximately 9 grams of fat and 3 grams of fiber per serving.

Gluten Free Banana Pancakes

4 Servings

An easy GP-friendly and gluten-free way to start the day!

Ingredients

- 1 cup gluten-free all-purpose flour

- 3 teaspoons baking powder

- 1 teaspoon cinnamon

- 1/2 teaspoon salt

- 2/3 cup unsweetened almond milk

- 1/4 cup unsweetened applesauce

- 1 tablespoon canola oil

- 3 teaspoons vanilla extract

- 3 ripe medium bananas, mashed

Directions

Preheat griddle. In a large bowl, combine flour, baking powder, cinnamon, and salt. In another bowl, whisk almond milk, applesauce, oil, and vanilla until combined. Add the wet ingredients to the dry ingredients and stir gently, just until moistened. Do not overmix. Fold in the bananas.

Coat griddle with nonstick cooking spray. Pour ¼ cupfuls on to griddle. When bubbles form on top and the sides start to set, gently flip. Cook 2-3 minutes on second side or until golden brown.

Approximately 4 grams of fat and 2 grams of fiber per serving. Wheat free. Milk free.

Pumpkin Spice Cream of Rice

1 Serving

I could've called this "Fall in a Bowl." That's what it tastes like: warm and pumpkiny and cinna-mony. You can substitute any kind of hot cereal that you like and can tolerate; simply use the cooking times and instructions on the package.

Ingredients

- 1/4 cup Erewhon Brown Rice Cream

- 1/2 cup unsweetened almond milk (or dairy, soy, or rice milk)

- 1/2 cup water

- 1/4 cup solid pack pumpkin

- 1 tablespoon smooth almond butter

- Maple syrup, to taste

- Cinnamon or pumpkin pie spice, to taste

Directions

Put rice cereal into a small saucepan. Slowly add milk and water, stirring constantly. Bring to a boil over high heat. Reduce heat and simmer for 3 minutes. Remove from heat. Stir in all other ingredients.

Approximately 8 grams of fat and 3 grams of fiber per serving. Wheat free. Milk free.

Live Well Tip: Have a Hot Breakfast

Since it's low in fat, low in fiber, and easy to digest, hot cereal is often very well tolerated by GPers. There are tons of possible flavor combinations; mix and match to find your favorites! Cooking times vary for each type of cereal, so prepare according to the directions on the package. Prepared individual portions can be frozen in plastic containers for a quick and easy meal.

Choose a Cereal:

- Cream of Wheat—good source of iron; low in fiber

- Cream of Rice/Brown Rice Cream—gluten free; low in fiber

- Cream of Buckwheat—gluten free; low in fiber

- Quinoa Flakes—gluten free; higher protein; 2.6 g fiber

Choose a Liquid:

- Water

- Low-fat milk (dairy, almond, rice, soy, or coconut)

- Juice (apple, white grape)

- Broth (for savory versions)

Choose Add-Ins:

- 1/4–1/2 cup homemade applesauce

- 2–4 ounces fruit puree (or baby food)

- 1/2 banana, mashed up

- 1/4 cup canned pumpkin

- 1/4 cup mashed sweet potatoes

- 1–2 tablespoons PB2

- 2 tablespoons GPNB (see page 148)

- 1 tablespoon smooth almond butter, creamy peanut butter or Nutella

- 1 scoop of protein powder, any flavor

- Honey or maple syrup

- Jelly or seedless jam

- Cinnamon, ginger, apple pie spice, or pumpkin pie spice

- Parmesan cheese (for savory versions)

5 Minute Breakfast Sandwich

2 Servings

A portable, couldn't-be-faster breakfast with a GP-friendly balance of protein, fat, and carbohydrates. If you tolerate animal protein, you can also add a slice of Canadian bacon.

Ingredients

- 2 eggs

- 2 English muffins

- 2 slices reduced-fat Colby Jack cheese

Directions

Toast English muffins. Meanwhile, heat a nonstick skillet over medium-low heat. Lightly beat eggs and pour into preheated skilled to scramble. Sprinkle 2 tablespoons of shredded cheese on the bottom half of each toasted muffin and divide the scrambled eggs between the two. Cover with the tops of the English muffins.

Approximately 8 grams of fat and 1 gram of fiber per serving.

Nutty Banana Waffle

1 Serving

Frozen waffles aren't that exciting and they're not that nutritious, either. But we're dressing them up with nutrient-dense nut butter and potassium-rich bananas in this simple weekday breakfast.

- 1 frozen waffle, such as Van's Totally Natural Minis

- 1 tablespoon nut butter

- 1/2 banana, sliced

- Maple syrup, to taste

Toast waffle according to directions. Spread hot waffle with nut butter and top with sliced banana. Drizzle with maple syrup, if desired.

Approximately 9 grams of fat and 2 grams of fiber per serving.

Easy Baked Eggs

4 Servings

Protein-rich and full of nutrients, serve alongside a thick slice of sourdough toast and a glass of fresh juice for an easy but satisfying breakfast.

Ingredients

- 4 large organic, free-range eggs

- 1/2 teaspoon freshly ground black pepper

- 1/2 teaspoon salt

- 4 teaspoons fat-free half-and-half or non-dairy milk

Directions

Preheat oven to 350°F. Spray each of 4 (6-ounce) ramekins with canola oil spray. Break 1 egg into each prepared ramekin. Sprinkle eggs evenly with pepper and salt; spoon 1 teaspoon milk over each egg. Place ramekins in a 13 x 9-inch baking dish; add hot water to pan to a depth of 1 ¼ inches. Bake for 25 minutes or until eggs are set.

Approximately 5 grams of fat and 0 grams of fiber per serving. Wheat free.

Live Well Tip: Make a batch of GPNB (GPers' Nut Butter)

I love nut butter. It's nutrient-rich, satisfying, great for balancing blood sugar, and...well...just really tasty. But it's also fairly high in fat. And while up to two tablespoons per day is typically well tolerated as part of a GP-friendly diet, sometimes it's nice to have a little more wiggle room. Enter GPNB! The GPers Nut Butter: all of the flavor, half the fat...

Ingredients

- 3/4 cup natural nut butter (peanut butter, almond butter, cashew butter, etc.)

- 3/4 cup unsweetened vanilla almond milk

- I tablespoon pure maple syrup or honey

- I/4 teaspoon ground cinnamon (optional)

Directions

Add almond milk, nut butter, maple syrup and honey (and cinnamon, if desired) to a blender in that order. Blend until smooth. Store in the refrigerator in a tightly sealed container.

Approximately 4 grams of fat and 0.5 gram of fiber per tablespoon. Wheat free. Milk free.

Gluten Free Banana Muffins

12 Servings

Whether you have celiac disease or you're just sensitive to wheat (I notice a lot more bloating when I eat too much wheat), these gluten-free muffins are a really tasty alternative.

Ingredients

- 1 cup mashed ripe bananas
- 2 tablespoon coconut oil
- 2 tablespoon applesauce
- 1 cup organic light brown sugar
- 2 teaspoon vanilla extract
- 2 eggs
- 1/4 teaspoon lemon juice
- 1 cup sorghum flour
- 1/2 cup potato starch (not potato flour!)
- 1 teaspoon baking soda
- 1 teaspoon baking powder
- 1/4 teaspoon salt
- 1-1/2 teaspoons xanthan gum
- 1 teaspoon cinnamon

Directions

Preheat your oven to 375°F. Lightly spray a 12-muffin pan with cooking spray or line with paper liners. In a large bowl, combine the ingredients from bananas through lemon juice. In a separate bowl, combine the ingredients from sorghum flour through cinnamon. Add the dry ingredients into the banana mixture, stirring until well combined. Spoon the batter into the prepared muffin cups. Let sit for 20–30 minutes, and then bake in the center of a preheated oven for about 16 minutes. Let cool for 5 minutes, then remove from pan and cool completely on a wire rack.

Approximately 3 grams of fat and 2 grams of fiber per serving. Wheat free. Milk free.

Really Good Banana Muffins

12 Servings

I'm not usually a fan of low-fat banana muffins. They're usually too dry, tough, or flavorless. Not these! Give 'em a try. I bet you'll say, "These are really good banana muffins!"

Ingredients

- 2 cups all-purpose flour

- 3/4 cup granulated sugar, divided

- 1 teaspoon baking powder

- 1 teaspoon baking soda

- 1/4 teaspoon salt

- 3 tablespoons butter, softened

- 1 large egg

- 1 egg white

- 3 very ripe bananas, mashed

- 1/2 cup low-fat buttermilk

- 1/2 teaspoon vanilla extract

- 1/2 teaspoon banana extract (or just increase vanilla to 1 full teaspoon)

- 1/4 cup turbinado sugar (optional)

Directions

Preheat oven to 350 °F. Spray a muffin tin with nonstick cooking spray.

In a medium bowl, combine flour, ¼ cup sugar, baking powder, baking soda, and salt. Set aside. In another medium bowl, mash bananas, and then mix in extracts and buttermilk. Set aside. In a mixing bowl, beat together remaining sugar (1/2 cup) and softened butter until light and fluffy, about 2 minutes. Add egg and egg white, mixing until well combined. Turn the mixer to low and add about one-third of the banana mixture. Let mix until just combined. Add half of the dry ingredients. Repeat, ending with banana mixture. Mix until just combined. Do not over mix.

Scoop batter into prepared muffin tin. Sprinkle each muffin top with 1 teaspoon of turbinado sugar, if desired. Bake for 17–20 minutes, until muffins spring back when touched. Do not over bake. Allow to cool on a wire rack for about 10 minutes before removing from pan.

Approximately 3.5 grams of fat and 1 gram of fiber per serving.

Cheddar Cheese Scones

8 Servings

These cheesy scones pair well with an egg for breakfast or with a low-fat veggie soup for lunch or dinner.

Ingredients

- 2 cups all-purpose flour

- 1 tablespoon baking powder

- 2 teaspoon sugar

- ¼ teaspoon salt

- 3 tablespoon chilled butter, cut into small pieces

- 1 cup reduced-fat cheddar cheese

- ¾ cup fat-free buttermilk

- 2 large egg whites

Directions

Preheat oven to 400°F. Coat a baking sheet with nonstick cooking spray. Combine first four ingredients in a large bowl. Cut in butter with two knives or a pastry blender until crumbly. Add cheese. In a separate bowl, combine egg whites and buttermilk. Add milk mixture to flour mixture, stirring until moist. Turn dough onto a lightly floured surface and knead 5 times. Place dough on baking sheet and form into an 8-inch circle. Cut into 8 wedges without cutting all the way through the dough. Bake for 20 minutes or until lightly browned. Cool completely, then separate wedges.

Approximately 5 grams of fat and 1 gram of fiber per serving.

Lunch & Dinner

When walking, walk. When eating, eat.

–Zen proverb

Baked Risotto Cakes

4 Servings (2 cakes each)

These crispy little cakes are something I'd choose to eat even if I didn't have gastroparesis. True comfort food!

Ingredients

- 1 large egg

- 2 cups cold leftover risotto (see page 191)

- 1 cup panko bread crumbs, divided

Directions

Preheat your oven to 400°F. Lightly beat egg in a large bowl. Stir in the risotto and ½ cup bread crumbs. Form the mixture into 8 small cakes, using about ¼ cup mixture for each. Place the remaining ½ cup bread crumbs in a shallow dish. Coat each cake with bread crumbs.

Spray a large nonstick baking sheet with cooking spray. Arrange the cakes in a single layer and bake for 15 minutes. Flip cakes over and bake for another 10 minutes until golden brown.

Approximately 4.5 grams of fat and 1.5 grams of fiber per serving.

GP-Friendly Pigs in a Blanket

8 Servings (3 pieces each)

Hot dogs aren't something that most of us would consider GP-friendly, but the poultry hot dogs from Applegate Farms definitely are. Wrapped up in a doughy blanket, these go over well at casual get-togethers.

Ingredients

- 8 organic low-fat chicken or turkey hot dogs (such as Applegate Farms)

- 2-1/2 cups reduced-fat baking mix, either regular or gluten free

- 3/4 cup unsweetened plain almond milk

- Canola oil spray

Directions

Preheat the oven to 450°F. Spray a baking sheet with canola oil spray. Cut each hot dog into 3 pieces. In a medium-sized bowl, combine the baking mix and the almond milk. Knead the dough about 10 times. Take a small piece of dough and wrap it around one hot dog piece. Repeat until all hot dogs are wrapped with dough. Bake about 10 minutes or until golden brown.

Approximately 4.5 grams of fat and 1 gram of fiber per serving.

Egg Salad for One

1 Serving

Packed with protein, this makes an energizing lunch served either on sandwich bread or on a toasted English muffin. Or serve with crackers for a well-balanced snack.

Ingredients

- 1 whole peeled hard-boiled organic egg, chopped

- 2 peeled hard-boiled organic eggs (whites only), chopped

- 2 tablespoons 0% plain Greek yogurt

- 1 tablespoon reduced-fat mayonnaise

- Kosher salt and freshly ground black pepper, to taste

Directions

Gently mix all ingredients together in a small bowl.

Approximately 6 grams of fat and 0 grams of fiber per serving.

Three-Cheese Pitza

4 Servings

Pita Pizzas = Pitzas, an easy, all-in-one meal that's GP-friendly and family-friendly. This basic version is a great template for all kinds of variations: add sautéed mushrooms, steamed spinach, or diced chicken breast. Whatever works for you!

Ingredients

- 4 6-inch pitas

- 3/4 cup fat-free ricotta cheese

- 1/4 cup Parmesan cheese

- 1 teaspoon Italian seasoning

- 3/4 cup shredded reduced-fat mozzarella cheese

Directions

Preheat oven to 350°F. Stir Italian seasoning and Parmesan cheese into ricotta cheese. Top each pita with about ¼ cup ricotta cheese mixture. Sprinkle with 3 tablespoons mozzarella cheese. Place on ungreased baking sheet. Bake for 10–15 minutes until cheese is melted and pita is slightly browned.

Approximately 5 grams of fat and 1 gram of fiber per serving.

Roasted Red Pepper Pitza

4 Servings

Pitzas are great for family nights or social get-togethers. Everyone can choose their own toppings and variations. This particular version has the added nutrition boost and unique flavor of roasted red peppers. Adults—even non-GPers—love it!

Ingredients

- 4 6-inch pitas

- 1/2 cup fat-free ricotta

- 1/2 cup roasted red peppers

- 3/4 cup shredded reduced-fat mozzarella cheese

Directions

Preheat oven to 350°F. Puree roasted red peppers and ricotta cheese in a food processor or blender until smooth. Top each pita with about ¼ cup pepper/cheese mixture. Sprinkle each pita with 3 tablespoons mozzarella cheese. Place on ungreased baking sheet. Bake for 10–15 minutes until cheese is melted and pita is slightly browned.

Approximately 4 grams of fat and 2 grams of fiber per serving.

Pumpkin Pasta

4 Servings

This autumnal dish is dairy free, gluten free, vegan and GP-friendly. It's hard to believe how good it tastes! If you tolerate wheat, you can substitute white pasta for the brown rice pasta.

Ingredients

- 1 teaspoon olive oil
- 1 shallot (if tolerated), minced
- 1/2 cup pumpkin puree (canned)
- 1 cup vegetable broth
- 1/4 cup water
- 1/4 cup plain rice milk
- 1/2 teaspoon ground nutmeg
- 1/2 teaspoon dried parsley
- Salt and pepper, to taste
- 1/2 pound brown rice pasta

Directions

In a large saucepan, heat oil over medium heat. Cook shallot until soft, about 2 minutes. Add pumpkin, broth, water, rice milk, and spices. Stir until combined. Bring to a simmer and cook, stirring occasionally, for 10 minutes. Meanwhile, boil pasta according to package directions. Drain the pasta, reserving 1 cup of cooking water. Add pasta to the sauce and stir to coat. If sauce is too thick, add cooking water until desired consistency is reached.

Approximately 1.5 grams of fat and 1.5 grams of fiber per serving. Wheat free. Milk free.

Roasted Red Pepper Pasta

4 Servings

Many GPers find it difficult to tolerate tomato pasta sauce, probably due to its acidity. This roasted red pepper pasta is the answer. Packed with both flavor and nutrition, it's a great way to get more "red" into your diet. Substitute brown rice pasta for the penne if you're avoiding wheat.

Ingredients

- 8 ounces uncooked penne pasta *white pasta*
- 1 teaspoon olive oil
- 1 (7 ounce) jar roasted red peppers, drained
- 3/4 cup organic chicken broth
- 3/4 cup fat-free half-and-half or plain unsweetened almond or soy milk
- 4 teaspoons dried basil
- 1/2 teaspoon garlic salt (or sea salt)
- 2 teaspoons cornstarch
- 4 tablespoons shredded Parmesan cheese

Directions

Cook pasta in boiling water according to the directions on the package. Meanwhile, heat a large skillet over medium heat. Sauté roasted red peppers in olive oil for about 1 minute. Add the broth, ½ cup half-and-half or milk, basil, and salt to the skillet. Bring to a boil, then reduce heat and simmer for about 3 minutes, until thickened. Remove from heat and transfer to a blender or food processor. Process until smooth, then return to the pan. Stir together cornstarch and remaining milk. Slowly pour mixture into the skillet. Bring back to a boil and simmer for 2 more minutes, until thickened. Add cooked, drained pasta to the sauce. Sprinkle each serving with 1 tablespoon of Parmesan cheese.

Approximately 3 grams of fat and 2 grams of fiber per serving.

Live Well Tip: Stock Your Pantry

A well-stocked pantry makes preparing a variety of gastro-paresis-friendly meals less time consuming and therefore more appealing. Below is a list of the non-perishable items that most GPers will likely want to have on hand. Your staples may vary, of course, depending on your personal tolerances and preferences.

Canned/Boxed Goods

- Almond milk (unsweetened)

- Applesauce (no sugar added)*

- Baby food: assorted fruits and vegetables*

- Broth: beef, chicken, vegetable—without MSG

- Canned fruits: peaches, pears*

- Orgain (or other meal replacement drinks)

- Purees: butternut squash, sweet potato, pumpkin (solid pack)

- Rice milk *No diabetes*

- Soup: i.e. Imagine Foods Organic Creamy Soups

Grains

- Flour: unbleached all-purpose white flour or gluten free all-purpose flour blend

- Hot cereal: i.e. Erewhon Brown Rice Cream, Pocono Cream of Buckwheat, Quinoa Flakes

- Panko bread crumbs

- Pasta: white (made from wheat flour) or brown rice

- White rice: short grain (for pudding and risotto), long grain (to be used as a side dish)

Condiments/Miscellaneous

- Blackstrap molasses*

- Canola oil

- Cocoa powder (unsweetened)

- Cooking spray

- Ground cinnamon

- Ground ginger

- Honey or maple syrup (not pancake syrup)

- Nut butters: creamy almond butter, cashew butter and/or peanut butter*

- Olive oil (extra-virgin)

- Sea salt

- Sugar (granulated)

- Spices: based on preferences and tolerances

Easy Tuna Burgers

2 Servings

Tuna is a fantastic source of protein and is well tolerated by many GPers. This is a more interesting twist on the typical tuna sandwich. Make sure that your tuna is packed in water, not oil.

Ingredients

- 1 (6 ounce) can water-packed tuna, drained
- 1/4 cup bread crumbs
- 1 large egg
- 1 teaspoon Worcestershire sauce
- 1/4 teaspoon Old Bay seasoning
- 2 English muffins, split and toasted

Directions

Preheat a nonstick skillet over medium heat. Combine tuna, bread crumbs, egg, Worcestershire sauce, and salt in a medium bowl until well mixed. Shape into 2 patties. Spray skillet lightly with canola oil spray and grill patties about 4 minutes on each side. Serve each patty on an English muffin.

Approximately 6 grams of fat and 1 gram of fiber per serving.

Crusted Halibut

Four Servings

This ready-in-a-hurry dish can be made with any white fish. Serve with Herbed Couscous and a GP-friendly veggie for a simple but satisfying meal.

Ingredients

- 1 pound halibut fillet, cut into 4 pieces

- 3 tablespoons flour

- 3 teaspoons lemon juice

- 2 teaspoons canola oil

- 1 teaspoon Italian seasoning

- 1/4 teaspoon salt

Directions

Preheat oven to 500°F. Spray a large baking dish with cooking spray. In a shallow bowl, combine flour, lemon juice, canola oil, Italian seasoning, and salt. Spread mixture on the top only of each piece of fish and place in baking dish. Bake until the fish is lightly browned, about 10 minutes.

Approximately 4 grams of fat and less than 1 gram of fiber per serving. Milk free.

Breaded Chicken Cutlets

4 Servings

Basic but delicious. If you tolerate poultry, it doesn't get much easier than this.

Ingredients

- 1 egg

- 4 skinless, boneless chicken breast cutlets

- 1/2 cup panko bread crumbs

- 1 teaspoon dried sage

Directions

Preheat oven to 375°F. Line a baking sheet with parchment paper or spray with nonstick cooking spray. Lightly beat egg in a small shallow bowl. Combine sage and bread crumbs in a separate shallow bowl. Dip each cutlet into the egg and then into the bread crumb mixture. Place on baking sheet. Bake until chicken is cooked through and outside is crispy, about 15 minutes.

Approximately 2 grams of fat and less than 1 gram of fiber per serving. Milk free.

GP-Friendly Chicken Parmesan

4 Servings

This is a family-friendly dish that everyone will love. I've been feeding it to my husband for years! If you don't tolerate tomato sauce, leave it off of your piece.

Ingredients

- 1/4 cup grated fresh Parmesan cheese

- 1/4 cup panko breadcrumbs

- 1 teaspoon Italian seasoning

- 1/2 teaspoon dried basil

- 1/4 teaspoon salt, divided

- 1 large egg white, lightly beaten

- 1 pound chicken breast tenders

- 1 tablespoon butter

- 1 cup smooth (or strained) tomato sauce

- 1/3 cup shredded reduced-fat mozzarella cheese

Directions

Preheat oven to 350°F. In a shallow dish, combine Parmesan cheese, breadcrumbs, and seasonings. In a separate dish, lightly beat egg white. Dip each chicken tender in egg white and then dredge in breadcrumb mixture. Melt butter in a nonstick skillet over medium heat. Add tenders and cook for 2-3 minutes on each side until browned. Place tenders in a baking dish. Cover evenly with sauce then sprinkle with mozzarella cheese and remaining Parmesan cheese. Bake for 20 minutes or until chicken is done and cheese is melted and bubbly.

Approximately 6 grams of fat and less than 1 gram of fiber per serving.

Honey Mustard & Pretzel Chicken Tenders

4 Servings

Tangy, crispy and GP-friendly. What more can I say? Kids love these!

Ingredients

- 2 cups salted pretzel sticks or nuggets

- 1/3 cup honey Dijon mustard

- 2 tablespoons milk or water

- 1 pound skinless chicken tenders

Directions

Heat oven to 375°F. Pulse pretzels in a food processor (or crush by hand) to make crumbs. Combine mustard and milk or water in a small bowl. Dip each tender in the mustard mixture, shaking off excess, then coat with pretzel crumbs. Place on baking sheet. Bake 15 minutes or until cooked through and crispy on the outside.

Approximately 4 grams of fat and 1 gram of fiber per serving.

Venison Meat Loaf

8 Servings

Wild game is lower in fat than beef and may be well tolerated, especially when ground. One 3-ounce serving of ground venison contains only about 2 grams of fat but a whopping 26 grams of protein! Even those who don't care for venison are likely to enjoy this flavorful, moist meatloaf.

Ingredients

- 2 eggs

- 8 ounces strained tomato sauce

- 1 shallot (if tolerated), finely chopped

- 1 cup dry bread crumbs

- 1-1/2 teaspoons salt

- 1/8 teaspoon pepper

- 1-1/2 pounds ground venison

- 2 tablespoons brown sugar

- 2 tablespoons brown mustard

- 1 tablespoon apple cider vinegar

Directions

Preheat oven to 350 °F. Lightly beat eggs in a large bowl. Add tomato sauce, shallots, bread crumbs and spices. Add venison and mix well. Press into an ungreased 9 x 5-inch loaf pan. Combine brown sugar, mustard, and vinegar in a small bowl. Spread over top of loaf. Bake uncovered for about 70 minutes or until a meat thermometer reads 160°.

Approximately 4 grams of fat and 1 gram of fiber per serving.

Side Dishes

Good food is wise medicine.

–Alison Levitt, M.D.

Creamy Cauliflower

4 Servings

Need a break from potatoes? Cauliflower makes excellent "faux" mashed potatoes. While cauliflower isn't GP-friendly when eaten whole, it's often well tolerated when pureed.

Ingredients

- 1 head of cauliflower, florets only

- 1/2 cup 0% plain Greek yogurt

- 1/4 cup grated Parmesan cheese

- 1/4 cup chicken broth

- Salt and pepper, to taste

Directions

Fill a medium pot with water and bring to a boil over high heat. Add cauliflower florets and cook for 8–10 minutes or until soft. Drain. In a food processor, combine the cauliflower, Greek yogurt, and Parmesan cheese. Puree until creamy. Add chicken broth, a tablespoon at a time, until the desired consistency is reached. Add salt and pepper to taste.

Approximately 1 gram of fat and 2 grams of fiber per serving. Wheat free.

Parmesan Potato Fries

8 Servings

If you miss french fries, you've got to try these. You won't believe they're GP-friendly!

Ingredients

- 4 large baking potatoes, peeled
- 1 tablespoon olive oil
- 1/4 cup grated Parmesan cheese
- 1 teaspoon salt

Directions

Preheat oven to 425°F. Line a baking sheet with heavy-duty foil. Cut each potato into thin french-fry shaped pieces. Put potatoes, olive oil, Parmesan cheese and salt into a bowl and toss to coat. Arrange in single layer on baking sheet. Bake for 30–40 minutes or until tender inside and crispy outside.

Approximately 2 grams of fat and 2 grams of fiber per serving. Wheat free.

Brown Sugar Beets

6 Servings

If you find the taste of beets too "earthy," give this glazed version a try. Beets are an excellent source of folate, manganese, and potassium.

Ingredients

- 3 tablespoons dark brown sugar

- 2 tablespoons orange or apple juice

- 1 tablespoon unsalted butter

- 1/4 teaspoon salt

- 3 cups beets, cut into ½-inch cubes

Directions

Trim greens and root ends from beets. Peel with a vegetable peeler. Cut into ½-inch cubes. Fill a pot with 1 inch of water. Place beets in a steamer basket in the pot and cover. Steam over high heat about 10–15 minutes, until tender.

Combine brown sugar, apple juice, butter, and salt in a large nonstick skillet. Cook over medium heat until the mixture has melted and starts to bubble. Stir in steamed beets and cook for 6–8 minutes, until most of the liquid has evaporated and the beets are coated with glaze. Serve warm.

Approximately 2 grams of fat and 2 grams of fiber per serving. Wheat free.

Creamed Spinach

2 Servings

Spinach is one of the few green vegetables that are GP-friendly. Pureeing the steamed spinach in this recipe increases the likelihood that it'll be well tolerated.

Ingredients

- 10 ounces fresh baby spinach

- 1 tablespoon water

- 2 teaspoons butter

- 1 tablespoon all-purpose flour

- 1/2 cup unsweetened almond milk

- 1/8 teaspoon ground nutmeg

- 1/8 teaspoon salt

- 1/8 teaspoon freshly ground pepper

- 2 tablespoons grated Parmesan cheese

Directions

Heat a large nonstick skillet over medium heat. Add spinach and water and cook for about 90 seconds, until spinach is wilted. Transfer to food processor and process until smooth.

In a small saucepan, melt butter over medium heat. Add flour and cook for about 30 seconds. Add milk, nutmeg, salt and pepper and cook about 1 minute, whisking constantly, until thickened. Add the spinach to the sauce. Stir in cheese and serve.

Approximately 3 grams of fat and 2 grams of fiber per serving.

Live Well Tip: Pureeing 101

Fruit and veggie purees can be served alone as side dishes or incorporated into other recipes, such as soups, smoothies, sauces, and more. Here's a quick primer on making purees:

Tools

- Rice cooker or a collapsible steamer and a medium pot with a lid

- Colander/strainer

- Hand-turned food mill, food processor, Magic Bullet, blender, or Vitamix

- Measuring cups

- Freezer-safe Ziploc bags and/or freezer-safe plastic food storage containers

Steps

- Prepare the fruits and vegetables by washing, peeling, and chopping them.

- Cook fruits and vegetables by steaming, baking or boiling them until fork tender. (If preparing a variety of purees, cook each fruit or veggie separately.)

- Drain the cooked fruits/veggies in a colander.

- Placed cooked fruits/veggies in food processor or blender and puree until smooth. (You may need to add a very small amount of water to some purees to get them to a smooth consistency.)

- Cool purees.

- Measure into ½-cup or ¼-cup portions and package in Ziploc bags or small food storage containers.

- Store purees in the freezer. (If you'll be using them within the next 2–3 days, put it in the fridge.)

Tips

- If boiling produce to soften it, use as little water as possible and add some of the cooking water back in while pureeing to retain the nutrients which can be lost during boiling.

- To prepare fresh beets or sweet potatoes, roast them in the oven (unpeeled and wrapped in aluminum foil) until easily pierced by a fork. Peel beets or scoop flesh out of sweet potato peel, add to processor and puree.

- You can use canned beets, peaches, pears, roasted red peppers, etc. for purees, if you'd like. No need to cook them first. Just open the can, dump it into the blender and puree.

- Grains like rice, quinoa, and millet can also be pureed or ground in a food mill. Cook them first according to package directions and then process.

Tangy Mashed Potatoes

8 Servings

A tangy twist on classic mashed potatoes, using chicken broth instead of butter and Greek yogurt in place of sour cream. Your family will never know that these are nearly fat free!

Ingredients

- 3 pounds peeled, diced Yukon Gold potatoes

- 6 ounces fat-free chicken broth, warmed in microwave

- 6 ounces 0% Greek yogurt

- 1 teaspoon salt

Directions

Fill a large pot with water. Add potatoes and bring to a boil. Cook for about 20 minutes or until tender. Drain well. Mash or put through a potato ricer, adding broth until desired consistency is reached. Stir in yogurt and salt.

Approximately 1 gram of fat and 2 grams of fiber per serving. Wheat free.

Rosemary Roasted Carrots

6 Servings

This is a simple but delicious side dish. Roasting the carrots at a high temperature intensifies the flavor and natural sweetness, which pairs well with the savory rosemary. All or some of the roasted carrots can be pureed in a food processor, if a soft dish desired.

Ingredients

- 1 pound carrots, peeled

- 2 teaspoons olive oil

- 1 teaspoon dried rosemary

- 1/2 teaspoon sea salt

Directions

Preheat oven to 450°F. Cut carrots into 1-inch pieces. Toss carrots with olive, rosemary, and salt until well coated. Spread onto a baking sheet lined with aluminum foil or place in a roasting pan. Roast about 25 minutes or until very soft and beginning to brown.

Approximately 1.5 gram of fat and 2 grams of fiber per serving. Wheat free. Milk free.

Gingered Butternut Squash

6 Servings

While butternut squash is fibrous, it's often well tolerated when pureed. This comforting dish combines the nutritional benefits of squash with the antiemetic properties of ginger. If you don't have fresh ginger on hand, substitute ½-1 teaspoon of ground ginger.

Ingredients

- 2 medium butternut squash, peeled, seeded and cubed

- 1 tablespoon butter

- 1 tablespoon maple syrup

- 1–2 tablespoons fresh ginger, finely grated (to taste)

- 3/4 teaspoon salt

- 1/4 teaspoon pepper

- 1/8 teaspoon ground nutmeg

- 2 tablespoons fat-free half-and-half

Directions

Place squash in a large saucepan. Cover with water. Bring to a boil over high. Cover, reduce heat, and simmer for 15 minutes or until tender. Drain well. Transfer to a food processor. Add butter and syrup. Process until smooth. Add in ginger, salt, pepper, nutmeg, and half-and-half, processing until well blended. Serve immediately.

Approximately 2 grams of fat and 3 grams of fiber per serving. Wheat free.

Minute Mashed Sweet Potatoes

4 Servings

This nutrient-packed side dish is literally ready in about a minute thanks to canned sweet potato puree.

Ingredients

- 1 15-ounce can organic sweet potato puree

- 3 tablespoons milk (any kind you tolerate)

- 1 tablespoon maple syrup

- 1/4 teaspoon cinnamon

- 1/4 teaspoon nutmeg

Directions

Heat sweet potato puree in the microwave or over the stovetop until warm. Stir in all other ingredients until well mixed. Serve immediately.

Approximately 0 grams of fat and 2 grams of fiber per serving. Wheat free.

Oven Roasted Vegetable Medley

4-6 Servings

Balsamic vinegar and walnut oil take this simple side dish to the next level. If you don't have those ingredients, simply use olive oil and leave out the vinegar. You'll still get lovely roasted veggies.

Ingredients

- 1 large sweet potato, peeled and cubed

- 1/2 pound baking potatoes, peeled and cubed

- 1/2 pound carrots, peeled and thickly sliced

- 1/2 pound turnips, peeled and cubed

- 6 ounces mushrooms, halved

- 1 tablespoon walnut oil

- 1/2 tablespoon balsamic vinegar

- 1 teaspoon salt

Directions

Preheat oven to 425°F. In a large roasting pan, combine vegetables, oil, vinegar, and salt. Roast for 35-40 minutes, or until vegetables are tender and lightly browned. Serve warm or at room temperature.

Approximately 4 grams of fat and 3 grams of fiber per serving. Wheat free. Milk free.

Maple Apple-Pear Sauce

8 Servings

For a twist on regular applesauce, try this naturally sweetened fruit puree. It makes a tasty side dish, dessert, or snack.

Ingredients

- 4 medium apples, peeled and coarsely chopped

- 1 medium pear, peeled and coarsely chopped

- 3/4 cup water

- 2 tablespoons maple syrup

- 1/2 teaspoon ground cinnamon

- 1/4 teaspoon ground nutmeg

Directions

Combine all ingredients in a large sauce over medium-high heat. Bring to a boil. Reduce heat to a simmer. Cover and cook 15-20 minutes or until very tender, stirring occasionally. Mash with a potato masher or puree in food processor until desired consistency. Serve warm or cold.

Approximately 0 grams of fat and 2 grams of fiber per serving. Wheat free. Milk free.

Basmati Rice with Turmeric and Mushrooms

4 servings

Turmeric is a brightly-colored spice with powerful anti-inflammatory properties.

Ingredients

- 1/2 tablespoon olive oil

- 2 cups organic, free-range chicken broth

- 1 cup basmati or jasmine rice

- 1/2 cup thinly sliced mushrooms

- 1/2 teaspoon turmeric

- Salt and pepper, to taste

Directions

Rinse the rice in a fine mesh strainer under cold water until water runs clear. Place rice in a large bowl, cover with water and let sit for 30 minutes before proceeding with the recipe. Heat oil in a medium saucepan over medium heat. Add rice and sauté for 2 minutes, stirring frequently. Add broth, mushrooms, and turmeric. Increase heat and bring to a boil. Reduce heat to low. Cover and simmer for 18–20 minutes, until broth is absorbed and rice is tender. Fluff with a fork before serving. Add salt and pepper to taste.

Approximately 2 grams of fat and 2 grams of fiber per serving. Wheat free. Milk free.

Herbed Couscous

4 servings

Couscous is perfect for busy evenings, since it takes just 5 minutes to cook. Using chicken broth instead of water imparts more flavor, as does toasting the couscous in olive oil prior to boiling.

Ingredients

- 1/2 tablespoon olive oil

- 1/4 cup finely chopped shallots (if tolerated)

- 1 cup uncooked white couscous

- 1 cup organic chicken broth

- 1 tablespoon flat-leaf parsley, finely chopped

- 1 teaspoon thyme, finely chopped

Directions

Heat a small saucepan over medium-high heat. Add oil to pan, swirling to coat. Add shallots; sauté 2 minutes or until tender. Stir in couscous; sauté 1 minute. Add broth and salt; bring to a boil. Cover, remove from heat, and let stand 5 minutes. Fluff with a fork. Stir in parsley and thyme.

Approximately 1.5 grams of fat and 2 grams of fiber per serving. Milk free.

Yellow Couscous

8 Servings

The squash puree in this recipe ups the nutrient quality and adds color to this tasty side dish.

Ingredients

- ½ cup vegetable broth

- 1 cup couscous

- ½ cup butternut squash puree

- 1 tablespoon butter

- 2 tablespoon grated Parmesan cheese

- ½ teaspoon salt

Directions

Bring broth to a boil over high heat in a medium saucepan. Remove from heat and stir in couscous, squash, butter, Parmesan cheese, and salt. Cover and let stand for about 7 minutes, until all liquid is absorbed.

Approximately 2 grams of fat and 1 gram of fiber per serving.

Easy Parmesan Risotto

4 Servings

This is a "cheater" version of risotto, which typically requires a lot of time, patience, and stirring. This GP-friendly version is quick, easy, and deliciously creamy! Make a double batch and use leftovers for Baked Risotto Cakes (page 157).

Ingredients

- 1/2 tablespoon butter or olive oil

- 2/3 cup uncooked Arborio rice

- 2 cups organic chicken stock

- 1/4 cup grated Parmesan cheese

Directions

Melt butter or heat oil in a medium saucepan over medium heat. Add rice and cook for 2 minutes, stirring frequently. Add broth. Bring to a boil. Reduce heat and simmer, covered, for 20 minutes. Do not lift the lid. Remove saucepan from heat and let stand, covered, for 5 minutes. Stir in Parmesan cheese and serve.

Approximately 3 grams of fat and 1 gram of fiber per serving. Wheat free.

Soups

Worries go down better with soup.

–Jewish proverb

Roasted Vegetable Stock

4 Servings

Use this nourishing and flavorful stock as a base for soups, a cooking liquid for rice, or to thin purees.

Ingredients

- 1 onion, unpeeled, quartered

- 4 carrots, cut into large pieces

- 3 celery ribs, cut into large pieces

- 2 parsnips, cut into large pieces

- 1 turnip, cut into large pieces

- 1 pound button mushrooms

- 7 cups water, divided

- 1 bay leaf

- 1 teaspoon dried marjoram

- 1 teaspoon dried thyme

- 1 teaspoon sea salt

- Pepper, to taste

Directions

Preheat oven to 450°F. Put onions, celery, carrots, turnips, and parsnips in a roasting pan. Roast for 15 minutes. Stir. Add mushrooms. Roast for 15 more minutes. Remove from oven and stir in 1 cup of cold water.

Carefully pour vegetable mixture into a large stockpot. Stir in 6 cups of cold water. Bring to a boil over high heat. Reduce heat and simmer, uncovered, for 90 minutes. Add bay leaf and spices. Simmer another 30 minutes. Remove from heat; add salt and pepper to taste. Let cool completely. Strain stock through a fine mesh strainer. Discard vegetables. Store stock in the refrigerator for up to a week.

Approximately 1 gram of fat and 0 grams of fiber per serving. Wheat free. Milk free.

Creamy Chicken & Rice Soup

4 Servings

Creamy and comforting, this soup is a meal in itself. Perfect for chilly fall days!

Ingredients

- 2 medium carrots, chopped

- 4 cups organic chicken broth

- 1/3 cup uncooked long-grain rice

- 3/4 teaspoon dried basil

- 1/4 teaspoon pepper

- 1/2 cup rice milk

- 2 tablespoons flour

- 3/4 pound boneless, skinless chicken breast, cooked and shredded

Directions

Combine broth, rice, carrots, basil, and pepper in a large stock pot over medium-high heat. Bring to a boil. Reduce heat to a simmer. Cover and cook for 20 minutes or until carrots and rice are tender.

In a small bowl, combine flour and rice milk until smooth. Add to soup. Bring to a boil. Cook, stirring frequently, for 2 minutes or until thickened. Add chicken and heat through.

Approximately 2 grams of fat and 2 grams of fiber per serving. Milk free.

Live Well Tip: Fill Your Freezer

When you're cooking dinner for your family, it can seem pointless or daunting to make a special meal just for you. While I recommend trying to incorporate GP-friendly entrees or side dishes into the family dinner, both to cut down on the work and so that you can join in the meal, it's not always realistic. If your symptoms are flaring up, for example, you may not be able to tolerate "real" food.

Fortunately, most GP-friendly soups freeze well, especially pureed ones. Set aside a few hours a week to make a batch or two of soup. Pre-portion the soup into 8–12 ounce containers, depending on the meal size that you tolerate and whether or not you tend to eat anything along with your soup. Allow each portion to cool thoroughly and then just stick the containers in the freezer. Over time you'll fill your freezer with a variety of choices, and a nourishing GP-friendly meal will never be more than a few minutes away.

By the way, you can do the same with smoothies, muffins, pitza toppings, pasta sauces, and more. Having a freezer stocked with pre-portioned, homemade GP-friendly foods and ingredients makes incorporating more variety and nutrition much easier.

Turkey Noodle Soup

2 Servings

A tasty twist on the classic, this soup uses turkey instead of chicken and is easy to make in small batches. Add any combination of veggies that you tolerate.

Ingredients

- 2 cups water

- 3/4 cup cubed cooked skinless turkey breast

- 1 large celery rib, cut in half

- 1 small shallot (if tolerated), finely chopped

- 1/2 teaspoon salt

- 1/8 teaspoon dried marjoram

- 1/8 teaspoon pepper

- 1 bay leaf

- 1 russet potato, peeled and sliced

- 2 large carrots, peeled and sliced

- 1/2 cup uncooked wide egg noodles (or any short brown rice pasta)

Directions

In a large saucepan, combine water, turkey, celery, shallot, spices, and bay leaf. Bring to a boil. Cover and reduce heat. Simmer for 10 minutes. Carefully remove celery. Add the potato, carrots, and noodles. Return to a simmer and cook for 20 minutes or until the potatoes are very tender. Carefully remove bay leaf and serve.

Approximately 3 grams of fat and 2 grams of fiber per serving. Milk free.

Harvest Chicken Stew

6 Servings

If you don't tolerate poultry, simply swap two peeled and diced medium potatoes for the chicken in this recipe and cook along with the other veggies to make a yummy vegetarian stew.

Ingredients

- 3 teaspoons extra-virgin olive oil, divided

- 1 pound skinless chicken breast tenders, cut into bite-size pieces

- 1 shallot (if tolerated), peeled and chopped

- 1 medium sweet potato, peeled and chopped

- 2 medium carrots, peeled and chopped

- 1/2 teaspoon dried rosemary

- 1/2 teaspoon salt

- 1/4 teaspoon freshly ground pepper

- 4 cups organic chicken broth

- 2 tart apples, peeled and chopped

Directions

Heat 2 teaspoons of oil in a large stock pot over medium heat. Add chicken and cook for about 4 minutes, until cooked through. Remove from pot. Add remaining 1 teaspoon of oil to the pot, along with shallot, sweet potato, carrots, and spices. Cook for about 5 minutes until veggies are softened. Add broth and apples. Bring to a boil over high heat. Reduce heat to a simmer. Cook until the veggies are very tender, about 10 more minutes. Return the chicken to the soup and serve.

Approximately 5 grams of fat and 3 grams of fiber per serving. Wheat free. Milk free.

Carrot, Parsnip & Ginger Soup

4 Servings

Parsnips pair nicely with the ginger in this recipe to produce a woodsy flavor and a lighter-colored soup. You can substitute all carrots if you prefer a sweeter flavor or a lower-fiber dish.

Ingredients

- 1/2 tablespoon olive oil

- 4 carrots, peeled and chopped

- 1 pound parsnips, peeled and chopped

- 1 shallot (if tolerated)

- Fresh ginger, about 1-inch piece, peeled and sliced

- 4 cups organic chicken or vegetable broth

- Sea salt and pepper, to taste

Directions

Heat olive oil in a large saucepan over medium heat. Add shallot and cook until softened, about 3 minutes. Add broth, carrots, parsnips, and ginger. Bring to a boil over high heat. Reduce heat and simmer, covered, for 20 minutes or until veggies are tender. Remove from heat and allow to cool slightly. Puree until smooth using an immersion blender or food processor.

Approximately 2 grams of fat and 3 grams of fiber per serving. Wheat free. Milk free.

Mushroom Lovers' Soup

6 Servings

Mushrooms are a good source of B vitamins, which are essential for the proper functioning of the GI tract. As always, if you don't tolerate shallots, just leave them out.

Ingredients

- 2 teaspoons extra-virgin olive oil

- 1-1/2 pounds mushrooms, thinly sliced

- 1 shallot (if tolerated), diced

- 3 tablespoons all-purpose flour

- 2 tablespoons paprika

- 2 tablespoons dried dill

- 4 cups organic reduced-sodium beef broth

- 2 cups skim, soy, or rice milk

- 1-1/2 pounds white potatoes, peeled and cut into ½-inch pieces

- 1/2 cup 0% Greek yogurt

- Salt, to taste

Directions

Heat oil in a heavy stock pot over medium heat. Add mushrooms and shallot. Sauté about 15 minutes, or until the mushrooms are very soft. Add flour, paprika, and dill. Stir for about 20 seconds to cook out the taste of the flour. Add broth, milk, and potatoes. Bring to a simmer and cook until the potatoes are fork tender, about 15 minutes. Remove from the heat and stir in Greek yogurt and salt to taste. Puree if desired.

Approximately 2 grams of fat and 2 grams of fiber per serving.

Winter Vegetable Soup

6 to 8 Servings

This is one of my personal favorites. Definitely add the Sourdough Croutons (page 205)!

Ingredients

- 6 cups organic chicken broth

- 2 teaspoons olive oil

- 1/2 shallot (if tolerated), diced

- 1/2 pound baby carrots (half of a 16-ounce bag)

- 1 large parsnip, peeled and chopped

- 2 small turnips, peeled and chopped

- 3 medium (or 6 small) potatoes, peeled and chopped

- ½-inch piece of fresh ginger, peeled

- 1 bay leaf

- Salt and pepper, to taste

Directions

Heat olive oil in a large pot over medium heat. Add shallot and cook until soft. Add broth, all veggies, ginger, and bay leaf. Heat to a boil. Reduce heat and simmer at least 30 minutes, until veggies are very soft. Fish out the bay leaf. Puree the soup in a food processor or blender until smooth. Add additional broth, if necessary, to achieve desired consistency. Season with salt and pepper to taste.

Approximately 2 grams of fat and 3 grams of fiber per serving. Wheat free. Milk free.

Live Well Tip: Add Croutons

Croutons are a great way to dress up a bowl of GP-friendly soup and add some crunch to an otherwise liquid meal. Though you can buy premade croutons, making your own is simple. Check out the recipe below. You can proportion individual servings into small Ziploc bags.

Sourdough Croutons

12 Servings (1/3 cup each)

Ingredients

- 4 cups day-old sourdough bread, cut into 1-inch cubes

- 1 tablespoon olive oil

- 1/2 teaspoon sea salt

- Pepper, to taste (optional)

Directions

Preheat oven to 325 °F. Toss bread cubes, olive oil, and seasonings in a large bowl to coat. Place in a single layer on baking sheet sprayed with nonstick cooking spray. Bake for about 20 minutes, until brown and crunchy.

Approximately 1.5 grams of fat and less than 1 gram of fiber per serving.

Ten Minute Butternut Squash Soup

6 Servings

Using canned butternut squash and baby food carrots makes this creamy soup very easy to prepare. You can substitute a can of solid pack pumpkin for the squash puree; it will raise the fiber content about 1.5 grams per serving.

Ingredients

- 1 15-ounce can organic butternut squash puree

- 2 4-ounce jars organic baby food carrots (or homemade carrot puree)

- 2 cups organic vegetable broth

- 1-1/2 cups plain rice milk

- 1/2 teaspoon grated nutmeg

- Salt and pepper to taste

Directions

Add squash puree, carrots, broth, rice milk, and nutmeg to a large pot. Bring to a simmer over medium heat and cook for about 10 minutes. Remove from heat and add salt and pepper to taste.

Approximately 1 gram of fat and 2 grams of fiber per serving. Wheat free. Milk free.

Slow Cooker Potato Dill Soup

6 Servings

Substitute whatever kind of milk you tolerate best in this flavorful set-it-and-forget-it soup.

Ingredients

- 6 large potatoes, peeled and cubed

- 4 cups chicken or vegetable broth

- 1 cup water

- 1/2 cup thinly sliced carrots

- 2 tablespoons butter

- 1/2 teaspoon celery salt

- 1/4 teaspoon pepper

- 2 tablespoons dried dill

- 1 cup skim, soy, or rice milk

Directions

In a large slow cooker combine the ingredients from potatoes through dill. Cover and cook on high for about 4-5 hours or on low for about 6-7 hours, or until the vegetables are tender (exact timing will vary depending on your slow cooker). Add milk, stirring well. Using an immersion blender, process to desired consistency—either chunky or completely pureed.

Approximately 4 grams of fat and 2 grams of fiber per serving. Wheat free.

Smoothies, Juices & Teas

Let food be thy medicine, thy medicine shall be thy food.

–Hippocrates

Live Well Tip: GP-Friendly Juicing

Juicing is one of the best ways to get more variety, nutrients, and healthy calories into your diet. You can drink the juice of nearly all fruits and vegetables, including ones that those of us with gastroparesis cannot eat whole. Though fresh juice is GP-friendly, it's important that you start with small amounts.

Here are some notes and tips to help you get the most out of juicing:

- Juicers come in a variety of price ranges. Centrifugal juicers tend to be less expensive than masticating juicers, which extract more juice. Either will work. Choose whichever best fits into your budget at this time.

- Almost any kind of fruit or vegetable can be juiced, though some are more difficult to digest than others. Leafy greens tend to be the most difficult to tolerate.

- Start by juicing each fruit and vegetable separately to test whether or not you tolerate it before experimenting with combinations.

- Use organic produce whenever possible.

- Peel and core all fruits and vegetables before putting them in the juicer.

- Anything that will not be peeled (berries, celery, spinach, etc.), should be washed thoroughly.

- Cut vegetables into pieces that can be fed through the juicer's feed tube easily.

- Feed soft fruit through the juicer first and follow with harder fruits/veggies.

- Strain juices through a fine mesh strainer to remove pulp. (I strain twice!)

- Serve juices immediately. Nutrients are lost as they are exposed to air.

- Too much juice is likely to upset your stomach. Start slowly with no more than 4–6 ounces of juice per day. Increase consumption as tolerated.

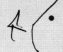
- Dilute juices with water—2 ounces for every 4 ounces of juice—to make them easier to digest.

- Dark vegetables have strong flavors. Dilute with an equal amount of water or more mild-flavored juices to make them more palatable.

- Clean the juicer as soon as possible after you make the juice to prevent residue from hardening.

Juices

These recipes require an electric juicer. All recipes make one to two servings of juice, depending on the quality of your juicer and your tolerances. Feed ingredients through machine in the order listed (except for honey, which should be stirred into the juice at the end). Strain juice through a fine mesh strainer to remove any pulp before drinking.

Carrot-Apple-Ginger Juice

- 2 large carrots, peeled and trimmed

- 2 apples*, peeled and cored

- ½-inch piece of gingerroot, peeled

Substitute 1 beet, peeled and trimmed, to up the "red" in your diet.

Veggie Delight

- 4 carrots, peeled and trimmed

- 2 celery stalks, washed and trimmed

- 1/4 cucumber, peeled

- Handful of baby spinach, washed (optional)

Berry Good Juice

- 1 cup strawberries, washed and trimmed

- 1 cup blueberries, washed

Pineapple Ginger Juice

- 1 cup pineapple chunks

- ½-inch piece of gingerroot, peeled

- Honey, to taste

Red Apple Juice

- 1 pomegranate, flesh only—seeds removed

- 2 apples, quartered

Live Well Tip: Make a Great Smoothie

- Use fresh, organic produce whenever possible.

- Protein powder can be added to any smoothie recipe.

- Always add liquids to the blender first, followed by fruit and other ingredients.

- Freeze your fruit or buy frozen fruit from the store. Frozen fruit makes for thicker smoothies.

- Cooked white rice can be used to thicken smoothies and increase calories.

- If you prefer thinner smoothies, add more liquid or do not freeze your fruit.

- Don't make your smoothies too big, especially if you have trouble with regurgitation.

- Sip smoothies very slowly to enhance digestion and prevent regurgitation.

- Serve immediately, or the smoothie will begin to separate. Smoothies do not keep well in the refrigerator.

- Individual portions of smoothies can be frozen in 8- or 12-ounce plastic containers. These make a good on-the-go snack. Simply wait for them to thaw, and drink (or eat with a spoon).

- Smoothies are best made in blenders. Food processors don't produce a smooth result.

- Wash your blender as soon as possible to prevent residue from sticking. Make sure container and blades are thoroughly cleaned after each use.

- If you're planning to make a lot of smoothies and other pureed items, a Vitamix is a fantastic investment for GPers.

Basic Smoothie Recipe

- 1/2 cup of plain or vanilla Greek yogurt

- 1/2 cup of juice, milk, or milk substitute

- 1 cup frozen fruit

- 1 scoop protein powder (optional)

Blend all ingredients until smooth. Add more liquid, if necessary, until smoothie reaches desired consistency.

Smoothies

Add ingredients to the blender in the order listed and process until smooth. All recipes make one serving unless otherwise noted.

Piña Colada Smoothie

- 1/4 cup of pineapple juice

- 1/2 cup water or milk

- 1 scoop vanilla protein powder

- 1 diced banana, frozen

- 1 teaspoon coconut extract

Sweet Banana Smoothie

- 6 ounces unsweetened vanilla almond milk

- 1/2 banana, sliced and frozen

- 1/2 medium sweet potato, baked, and peeled

- 1/2 cup ice (optional)

- 1/4 teaspoon cinnamon

Mango-Peach Protein Smoothie

- 1/2 cup diced mango, frozen (available in the frozen foods section of most supermarkets)

- 1/2 cup 0% Greek yogurt

- 1/2 cup peach nectar

Chocolate Covered Almond Smoothie

- 1/2 cup unsweetened chocolate almond milk

- 1 tablespoon unsweetened cocoa powder

- 1 tablespoon almond butter

- 1 banana, frozen

- 2 teaspoons agave nectar, honey, or maple syrup (optional)

- 1 dash cinnamon

Pomegranate Banana Smoothie (2 servings)

- 3/4 cup POM Wonderful 100% Pomegranate Juice

- 1/2 cup unsweetened almond milk

- 1 large banana, frozen

- 1 scoop vanilla protein powder (optional)

- 1 teaspoon honey or stevia sweetener

Milk & Honey

- 3/4 cup non-fat plain yogurt

- 1 ripe banana, sliced and frozen

- 1 tablespoon honey

- 1/2 teaspoon vanilla extract

Easy Being Green Smoothie

- 3/4 cup unsweetened almond milk

- 1 banana, frozen

- 1 cup spinach leaves

Chocolate Covered Banana

- ½ cup chocolate soy milk

- 1 banana, sliced and frozen

- 3 teaspoons unsweetened cocoa

- ¼ teaspoon cinnamon

Summer Melon Smoothie (2 servings)

- 1 cup honeydew melon, cubed

- 1 cup cantaloupe, cubed

- 3/4 cup organic low-fat vanilla yogurt

- 1/4 teaspoon vanilla extract

- 1/2 cup ice cubes

Spiced Apple Smoothie (2 servings)

- 1/2 cup apple juice, fresh if possible (juice of 2 apples)

- 1/4 teaspoon cinnamon

- 1 teaspoon grated fresh gingerroot

- 1 banana, sliced and frozen

Hot Drinks

All recipes make two servings unless otherwise specified.

Ginger Tea

- 1-inch piece of fresh ginger

- 2 cups water

- Honey, optional

Cut ginger into thin slices. Simmer in water for 15–20 minutes. Strain into two cups. Stir in honey to taste.

Extra-Strength Ginger Tea: Simmer ginger in water for 1 hour or until liquid is reduced by half. Strain into cup and add honey to taste.

Hot Gingersnap

- 1-1/2 cups apple juice

- 1 cinnamon stick

- 2 ginger tea bags

- 2 teaspoons maple syrup

In a small saucepan, combine juice and cinnamon stick. Bring to a boil, then reduce heat and simmer for 20 minutes. Remove from heat. Add teabags, cover, and let steep for 5 minutes. Remove tea bags and strain into two teacups. Stir 1 teaspoon of maple syrup into each cup.

Chai Tea

- 2 cups water

- 5 whole cloves

- 6 whole cardamom pods

- 3 whole black peppercorns

- 1 cinnamon stick

- 2 slices of ginger (¼-inch thick)

- 1/2–3/4 cup milk

- Maple syrup to taste

Bring water, spices, and ginger to a boil in a small pot. Lower heat and simmer, covered, for about 40 minutes. Add milk and heat until nearly boiling. Remove from heat and strain through a fine mesh strainer. Pour into cups and serve immediately.

Desserts & Treats

All I really need is love, but a little chocolate now and then doesn't hurt!

–Charles Schulz

Chocolate Angel Food Cake

12 Servings

This is the perfect dessert to serve to a crowd with mixed dietary tolerances. Most importantly, angel food cake is GP-friendly with almost no fat or fiber.

Ingredients

- 1/2 cup potato starch
- 1/4 cup cocoa
- 1-1/4 cups superfine sugar, divided
- 10 egg whites
- 1/4 teaspoon salt
- 1/2 teaspoon lemon juice

Preheat oven to 350°F. Sift potato starch, cocoa, and ¼ cup sugar together into a small bowl.

In a separate bowl, beat the egg whites on low speed, slowly adding salt and lemon juice. Increase the speed until egg whites form soft peaks. Start adding remaining sugar, 1 tablespoon at a time. Continue beating until the egg whites are glossy and stiff. Sift dry ingredients ¼ cup at a time over the whites, gently folding them in after each addition.

Gently spoon batter into an ungreased 10-inch tube pan. Place pan on the middle rack and bake for 45 minutes until the edges of the cake have pulled away from the side of the pan. Remove from oven and place the pan upside down on a wire rack or invert on the neck of a wine bottle. Allow to cool for one hour before removing from pan.

Approximately 0 grams of fat and 1 gram of fiber per serving. Wheat free. Milk free.

Birthday Cake

16 Servings

I went for five years without a birthday cake after I was diagnosed with gastroparesis. No more, thanks to this GP-friendly version of classic yellow cake with chocolate frosting. While I typically don't recommend using mixes that contain artificial ingredients, organic mixes and scratch cake recipes don't work as well with these low-fat adaptations. So, for rare occasions like birthdays, I say it's okay to make an exception!

Cake

- 1 box Betty Crocker SuperMoist yellow cake mix*

- 1 cup unsweetened applesauce

- 1 cup water

Frosting

- 4 ounces light cream cheese

- 2 cups powdered sugar

- 1/4 cup dark cocoa powder

- 1/2 teaspoon pure vanilla extract

- 1–2 tablespoons non-fat milk (optional)

Preheat oven to 350°F. Spray a 9 x 13-inch baking pan with nonstick cooking spray.

Combine cake mix, applesauce, and water in a mixing bowl. Beat at low speed until combined and then at medium speed for 2 minutes. Pour into prepared pan and bake for 25–30 minutes, until a toothpick inserted 2 inches from the edge comes out clean. Cool completely before frosting.

To prepare frosting, mix cream cheese and powdered sugar (1 cup at a time) in a mixing bowl until smooth. Add cocoa powder and vanilla extract and beat again until smooth. Add milk if necessary to achieve desired consistency. Spread evenly over cooled cake.

*Note that other brands of cake mix may contain 2–3 more grams of fat per serving. Check the nutrition panel!

Approximately 3 grams of fat and 1 gram of fiber per serving.

Crystal's Snickerdoodles

36 Cookies

These are so good that nobody will believe you when you tell them they're low-fat. Bring a plate to parties, picnics, or potlucks, and I guarantee people will be asking for the recipe.

Ingredients

- 1-3/4 cups all-purpose flour

- 1/2 teaspoon baking soda

- 1/2 teaspoon cream of tartar

- 3/4 cup sugar

- 1/4 cup butter, softened

- 1/4 cup pure maple syrup

- 1 teaspoon vanilla

- 2 large egg whites

- 3 tablespoons sugar

- 2 teaspoons ground cinnamon

Directions

Preheat oven to 375°F. Combine flour, baking soda, and cream of tartar in a bowl. Set aside. Beat butter and 3/4 cup of sugar in a large bowl until light and fluffy, about 2–3 minutes. Add the maple syrup, egg whites, and vanilla. Beat until well blended. Gradually add the flour mixture to the sugar mixture, beating just until incorporated. Combine the remaining 3 tablespoons of sugar and the cinnamon in a small bowl. Form dough into 1-inch balls (a melon baller or small cookie scoop works well). Roll each ball in cinnamon-sugar. Place balls

2 inches apart on a baking sheet sprayed with nonstick cooking spray. Flatten balls with a fork or the bottom of a glass. Bake 7 minutes, or until set but still soft.

Cool on baking sheet for about 5 minutes, and then move to wire racks to cool completely. Store in an airtight container.

Approximately 1.5 grams of fat and less than 0.5 gram of fiber per cookie.

Ginger Molasses Cookies

24 cookies

No butter? No oil? No worries. These cookies come out soft and flavorful despite having only 6 grams of fat in the entire batch. Factor in the ginger and it just might be the perfect GP-friendly cookie!

Ingredients

- 1 cup dark molasses

- 3/4 cup brown sugar, packed

- 1 teaspoon apple cider vinegar

- 1 egg

- 2-1/3 cups all-purpose flour

- 2 teaspoons baking soda

- 1-1/2 teaspoons ground ginger

- 1/2 teaspoon salt

Directions

Preheat oven to 350°F. Line two large cookie sheets with parchment paper. In a large bowl, add molasses, brown sugar, vinegar, and egg. Stir until combined. In another bowl, sift together flour, baking soda, ginger, and salt. Add dry ingredients to the molasses mixture. Stir until combined. Drop cookies by the tablespoon onto prepared baking sheets, about 2 inches apart. Bake for 12 minutes or until edges are golden and cookies are set. Remove from oven. Let cool for 5 minutes before removing from pan.

Approximately less than 0.5 gram of fat and less than 0.5 gram of fiber per cookie. Milk free.

Lemon White Chocolate Chip Biscotti

48 Servings

Biscotti are crunchy Italian cookies that tend to be quite low in fat. This particular recipe doesn't call for any butter or oil, leaving some wiggle room for the addition of white chocolate chips!

Ingredients

- ¾ cup granulated sugar

- 1 teaspoon pure vanilla extract

- ½ teaspoon pure lemon extract

- 2 large eggs

- 1-2/3 cups all-purpose flour

- ½ teaspoon baking soda

- ¼ teaspoon salt

- 1 cup white chocolate chips (I use SunSpire chocolate chips – half the fat of Nestlé's!)

Directions

Preheat oven to 300°F. Coat a baking sheet with nonstick cooking spray. Combine sugar, eggs, and extracts in a large mixing bowl and beat until blended. In a separate bowl, combine flour, baking soda, and salt. Gradually add flour mixture to egg mixture, beating until well combined. Stir in chocolate chips. Shape dough into two 12-inch logs, about 2-1/2 inches wide each, on prepared baking sheet. Bake for 35 minutes. Remove from oven and cool for 10 minutes. Cut each log into 24 pieces. Place cut sides down on baking sheet and return to oven for 12 minutes. Turn pieces over and bake an addition 12 minutes. Remove and cool completely.

Approximately 1 gram of fat and 0 grams of fiber per serving.

Cinnamon Sugar Tortilla Chips

8 Servings

I made these for a Super Bowl party a few years ago and they were the first thing to go. They taste like churros, only crispier and GP-friendly!

Ingredients

- 8 8-inch flour tortillas

- Water

- 1/4 cup sugar

- 2 teaspoon cinnamon

- Canola oil spray

Directions

Preheat oven to 400°F. Combine cinnamon and sugar in a small bowl. Brush one side of tortillas *lightly* with water (just enough so the cinnamon-sugar will stick). Sprinkle with cinnamon-sugar mixture. Cut each tortilla into 8 wedges. Arrange wedges in a single layer on a cookie sheet sprayed with cooking spray. Bake for 6–8 minutes or until crisp. (Keep a close eye on them; they burn easily.) Cool before serving.

Approximately 2 grams of fat and 1 gram of fiber per serving.

Honey & Cinnamon Frozen Yogurt

4 Servings

If you like Pinkberry Frozen Yogurt, you'll love this. It's true frozen yogurt, without the additives you'll find in the store-bought stuff. Plus, each serving packs about 12 grams of protein! If you don't own an ice cream maker, pour the mixture into popsicle molds and freeze for about 6 hours to make yogurt pops.

Ingredients

- 16 ounces 2% Greek Yogurt

- 1/4 cup honey

- 1/2 teaspoon cinnamon

Directions

Place all the ingredients in a bowl and whisk to combine. Pour the yogurt mixture into an ice cream maker and chill according to manufacturer's directions.

Approximately 2.5 grams of fat and 0 grams of fiber per serving. Wheat free.

Crispy Cocoa Bars

12 Servings

You can substitute almost any cereal when making these chewy treats. Experiment to find your favorite!

Ingredients

- 3 tablespoons butter

- 5-1/2 cups of Erewhon Gluten-Free Cocoa Crispy Brown Rice Cereal

- 10-ounce package of miniature marshmallows

Directions

Melt butter in a large saucepan over low-medium heat. Add marshmallows and stir until they're completely melted. Remove pan from heat and add cereal. Stir until well coated. Spread mixture into a 9 × 9-inch pan lightly coated with cooking spray.

Let set for 20 minutes and then cut into 12 squares.

Approximately 3 grams of fat and 0.5 grams of fiber per serving.

Banana "Ice Cream"

1 Serving

We've talked about the importance of maximizing nutrition in every meal and snack. This means having ice cream and frozen yogurt as occasional treats only—not as everyday meals or snacks. Fortunately, there's an alternative that's 100 percent natural, GP-friendly, and packed with nutrition. What's more, there's only one ingredient: a banana. Skeptical? I was, too. But I'm telling you, this stuff is good. It has the consistency of real soft-serve ice cream and a pleasant, not overwhelming, banana flavor.

Ingredients

- 1 banana, peeled, sliced and frozen

Directions

Place frozen banana slices into a food processor or Vitamix. Process for several minutes. Initially, the mixture will look like little pellets. Keep going until it looks like soft-serve ice cream.

Peanut Butter "Ice Cream" Variation: add 1 tablespoon PB2 powdered peanut butter and 2 tablespoons dairy or non-dairy milk OR add two tablespoons GPNB—then process as directed.

Approximately 1 gram of fat and 3 grams of fiber per serving. Wheat free. Milk free.

Dairy-Free Banana Rice Pudding

12 Servings (1/2 cup each)

This creamy rice pudding gets a nutritional boost from the addition of bananas.

Ingredients

- 1 cup basmati rice

- 2 cups water

- 1/2 teaspoon salt

- 3 cups plus 1 tablespoon unsweetened vanilla almond milk, divided

- 1/3 cup light brown sugar

- 1/2 teaspoon ground cinnamon

- 1 tablespoon cornstarch

- 2 ripe bananas

- 1 teaspoon vanilla extract

Directions

Combine rice, water, and salt in a medium saucepan and bring to a boil over medium-high heat. Reduce heat to low, cover and cook until all of the liquid is absorbed, about 45 minutes. Stir in 3 cups of almond milk, brown sugar, and cinnamon and bring to a simmer over low-medium heat. Cook, stirring occasionally, for 10 minutes. In a small bowl, combine cornstarch and remaining 1 tablespoon of almond milk. Stir until smooth and then add to the pudding. Continue cooking, stirring frequently, about 10 more minutes or until the pudding is thick. Remove from heat. Mash or puree the bananas. Add bananas and vanilla extract to the pudding and stir to combine. Transfer to a large bowl or into individual serving dishes. Cover with plastic wrap and refrigerate at least 2 hours.

Approximately 2 grams of fat and 1.5 grams of fiber per serving. Wheat free. Milk free.

Gooey Grilled Bananas

4 Servings

While not quite "health food," these gooey bananas certainly surpass traditional s'mores when it comes to nutrition.

Ingredients

- 4 medium unpeeled ripe bananas

- 4 tablespoons miniature marshmallows

- 4 tablespoons miniature chocolate chips (optional)

Directions

Cut banana peel lengthwise about 1/2 inch deep, leaving 1/2 inch of the peel intact at both ends. Open peel wider to form a pocket. Fill each with 1 teaspoon chocolate chips and 1 tablespoon marshmallows. Shape four pieces of heavy-duty aluminum foil around the bananas, forming little boats. Grill, covered, over medium heat for 5–10 minutes or until marshmallows melt and are golden brown. Or wrap In foil and bake in a 350 degree oven for 12–15 minutes.

Approximately 4 grams of fat and 3 grams of fiber per serving.

Cinnamon Apples

8 Servings

Stir into hot cereal or spoon a bit of this warm apple mixture over Honey & Cinnamon Frozen Yogurt (see page 233) for a truly delicious treat.

Ingredients

- 6 cups chopped peeled Granny Smith apple (about 2 pounds)

- 1/2 cup packed brown sugar

- 1/4 cup apple juice

- 1 teaspoon ground cinnamon

- 1/8 teaspoon ground nutmeg

- 1/8 teaspoon salt

Directions

Combine all ingredients in a large, heavy saucepan. Cover and cook over medium-low heat 45 minutes or until apples are tender, stirring occasionally. Let stand 5 minutes.

Approximately 0 grams of fat and 2 grams of fiber per serving. Wheat free. Milk free.

Brownies for Everyone

16 Servings

Why are these called Brownies for Everyone? Because they're GP-friendly, but everyone else will want to eat them, too. I've made these with regular and gluten-free brownie mix and the results are great either way. I've actually found Betty Crocker Gluten Free Brownie Mix to be one of the best tasting among all mixes, not just other gluten-free varieties.

Ingredients

- 1 (16 ounce) box of regular brownie mix or Betty Crocker Gluten Free Brownie Mix

- 1/2 cup unsweetened applesauce

- 1 egg

- 1/4 cup water

Directions

Preheat oven to 350°F. Spray the bottom of a 9 x 9-inch pan with nonstick cooking spray. Combine all ingredients in a bowl and stir until just combined. Don't over mix. Pour into prepared pan and bake for 30–32 minutes, until a toothpick inserted 2 inches from the edge comes out clean. Don't over bake.

Approximately 2 grams of fat and 1 gram of fiber per serving.

GLOSSARY

Common Acronyms

GES: gastric electrical stimulation *or* gastric emptying scan

GI: gastrointestinal

GP: gastroparesis

GPers: people who have been diagnosed with gastroparesis

FGID: functional gastrointestinal disorders

FGIMD: functional gastrointestinal and motility disorders

LES: lower esophageal sphincter

PCP: primary care provider

SIBO: small intestinal bacterial overgrowth

Key Terms

Antiemetic: medication that prevents or alleviates nausea and vomiting

Autonomic nervous system: part of your nervous system that controls involuntary actions

Bezoar: a hardened mass of undigested material (food or other fibers) most often found in the stomach

Chronic: persisting over a long period of time

Complementary medicine: treatments that do not fall within the scope of conventional medicine but are used in conjunction with medical treatment

Constipation: reduced frequency of bowel movements; difficulty passing stools

Digestive system: the digestive tract—mouth, esophagus, stomach, small intestine, colon, rectum, and anus—and other organs that help the body break down and absorb food

Digestion: the process of breaking down and absorbing food

Disorder: a disturbance in regular or normal function

Dysmotility: abnormal or absent contractions of the muscles in the gastrointestinal tract

Dyspepsia: pain or discomfort located in the upper abdomen

Endoscopy: procedure used to visually examine the upper GI tract with a tiny camera on the end of a long, flexible tube

Enteric nervous system: subdivision of the autonomic nervous system that is located within and directly controls the gastrointestinal system

Enterra Therapy: gastric electrical stimulation

Epigastric: upper abdominal region

Esophagus: the organ that connects the mouth to the stomach

FODMAPs: fermentable oligo-, di- and mono-saccharides and polyols; may contribute to symptoms in some patients with functional GI and motility disorders

Functional disorder: a disorder in which the normal functioning of an organ or system is impaired in the absence of structural abnormalities

Functional dyspepsia: also called non-ulcer dyspepsia; recurrent upper abdominal pain, fullness, and/or bloating without an identifiable cause or evidence of delayed gastric emptying

Gastric Electrical Stimulation: treatment that uses an implanted electrical device called a gastric neurostimulator to provide mild electrical stimulation to the lower stomach nerves

Gastritis: inflammation of the stomach

Gastroenterologist: a doctor who specializes in digestive diseases and disorders

Gastrointestinal: pertaining to the stomach and intestines

Gastrointestinal (GI) tract: mouth, esophagus, stomach, small intestine, large intestine, rectum, and anus; also called the digestive tract

Gastrostomy: surgical creation of an external opening into the stomach for nutritional support or compression

GP-friendly: conducive to managing gastroparesis; usually well tolerated by people with gastroparesis

Heartburn: pain or burning sensation in the chest, usually associated with reflux of gastric juice into the esophagus

Hypothyroidism: deficiency of thyroid activity

Idiopathic: unknown cause

Intestines: also known as the gut or bowels; consists of the small intestine and the large intestine

Jejunostomy: surgical formation of an opening through the abdominal wall into the small intestine for nutritional support

Malabsorption: impaired absorption of nutrients in the GI tract

Motility: ability of the digestive organs to propel their contents through the digestive tract

Motility specialists: Gastroenterologists who specialize in motility disorders, including gastroparesis

Neurologic: pertaining to the nervous system

Peristalsis: wormlike muscular contractions that move food through the digestive tract

Post-viral: following or caused by a viral infection

Prokinetic: medication that enhances gastrointestinal motility

Pylorus: region of the stomach that connects to the duodenum (the beginning of the small intestine)

Refractory: not improved by treatment

Reflux: backward flow of food or acid from the stomach to the esophagus

Regurgitation: backward flow of undigested food

Sublingual: route of administration by which drugs are absorbed into the blood through tissues under the tongue

Visceral hypersensitivity: enhanced perception of stimuli—even normal stimuli—within the gut

About the Author

Crystal Zaborowski Saltrelli is currently the only Certified Health Counselor specializing in gastroparesis management and one of very few health professionals with both personal and professional experience with the condition. Through health counseling programs, books, and her website, Crystal helps people worldwide learn to live (well!) with gastroparesis.

Crystal's interest in holistic health and nutrition began soon after she was diagnosed with idiopathic gastroparesis in 2004 at the age of 23. She went on to study health counseling and holistic nutrition at the Institute for Integrative Nutrition and became certified by the American Association of Drugless Practitioners in 2010. Crystal also holds a bachelor's degree in sociology from Dartmouth College.

In addition to her health counseling practice, Crystal is actively involved in the greater gastroparesis community, currently serving as Nutritional Specialist for the Gastroparesis & Dysmotility Foundation and promoting gastroparesis advocacy and awareness through the Digestive Health Alliance.

Crystal lives in western New York with her husband, Raymond. For more information about living well with gastroparesis or to contact Crystal, please visit her website at www.LivingWithGastroparesis.com.

cottage for protein
Atkins for protein bar

Orgain - meal replacement
PYOP turnip puree mashed
Papaya capsules - how much

Ginger Ale

Zevia Soda (Ginger Ale ck for Ginger

Avoid High Fructose Corn Syrup in Ginger Ale

Protein Powder

No Maltrodextrin or Polydextose

Made in the USA
San Bernardino, CA
24 July 2016